Photodynamic Therapy

Procedures in Cosmetic Dermatology
Series Editor: Jeffrey S. Dover MD FRCPC
Associate Editor: Murad Alam MD

Botulinum Toxin
Alastair Carruthers MABM BCh FRCPC FRCP(Lon) and
Jean Carruthers MD FRCS(C) FRC(OPHTH)
ISBN 1 4160 2470 0

Soft Tissue Augmentation
Jean Carruthers MD FRCS(C) FRC(OPHTH) and
Alastair Carruthers MABM BCh FRCPC FRCP(Lon)
ISBN 1 4160 2469 7

Cosmeceuticals
Zoe Diana Draelos MD
ISBN 1 4160 0244 8

Laser and Lights: Volume 1
Vascular • Pigmentation • Scars • Medical Applications
David J. Goldberg MD JD
ISBN 1 4160 2386 0

Laser and Lights: Volume 2
Rejuvenation • Resurfacing • Hair Removal • Treatment of Ethnic Skin
David J. Goldberg MD JD
ISBN 1 4160 2387 9

Photodynamic Therapy
Mitchel P. Goldman MD
ISBN 1 4160 2360 7

Liposuction
C. William Hanke MD MPH FACP and Gerhard Sattler MD
ISBN 1 4160 2208 2

Treatment of Scars
Kenneth A. Arndt MD

Chemical Peels
Mark Rubin MD

Hair Restoration
Dowling B. Stough MD and Robert S. Haber MD

Leg Veins
Tri H. Nguyen MD

Blepharoplasty
Ronald L. Moy MD

Face Lifting
Ronald L. Moy MD

Towards the prevention and treatment of the most common form of cancer affecting the most people worldwide – skin cancer

Towards the treatment of the most common skin condition affecting teenagers worldwide – acne

Towards the advancement of patient care in dermatology

Mitchel P. Goldman

PROCEDURES IN COSMETIC DERMATOLOGY

Series Editor: Jeffrey S. Dover MD FRCPC

Associate Editor: Murad Alam MD

Photodynamic Therapy

Edited by

Mitchel P. Goldman MD

Associate Clinical Professor of Dermatology/Medicine, University of California, San Diego;
Medical Director, La Jolla SpaMD, La Jolla, CA, USA

Series Editor

Jeffrey S. Dover MD FRCPC

Associate Professor of Clinical Dermatology, Yale University School of Medicine, Adjunct Professor of
Medicine (Dermatology), Dartmouth Medical School, Director, SkinCare Physicians of Chestnut Hill,
Chestnut Hill, MA, USA

Associate Editor

Murad Alam MD

Chief, Section of Cutaneous and Aesthetic Surgery, Department of Dermatology, Northwestern
University, Chicago, IL, USA

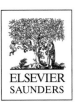

ELSEVIER
SAUNDERS

ELSEVIER
SAUNDERS

An imprint of Elsevier Inc.

First published 2005

ISBN: 1 4160 2360 7

British Library Cataloguing in Publication Data
A catalogue record for this book is available from the British Library

Library of Congress Cataloging in Publication Data
A catalog record for this book is available from the Library of Congress

---

Notice

Medical knowledge is constantly changing. Standard safety precautions must be followed, but as new research and clinical experience broaden our knowledge, changes in treatment and drug therapy may become necessary or appropriate. Readers are advised to check the most current product information provided by the manufacturer of each drug to be administered to verify the recommended dose, the method and duration of administration, and contraindications. It is the responsibility of the practitioner, relying on experience and knowledge of the patient, to determine dosages and the best treatment for each individual patient. Neither the Publisher nor the editor assumes any liability for any injury and/or damage to persons or property arising from this publication.

The Publisher

Printed in China
Last digit is the print number : 9 8 7 6 5 4 3 2 1

Commissioning Editors: **Sue Hodgson, Shuet-Kei Cheung**
Project Development Managers: **Martin Mellor Publishing Services Ltd, Louise Cook**
Project Managers: **Naughton Project Management, Cheryl Brant**
Illustration Manager: **Mick Ruddy**
Design Manager: **Andy Chapman**
Illustrators: **Richard Prime, Tim Loughhead**

Contents

Series Foreword   ix

Preface   xi

List of Contributors   xiii

1 Mechanism of Action of Topical Aminolevulinic Acid   1
Brian D. Zelickson

2 Treatment of Acne   13
Yoshiyasu Itoh

3 ALA-PDT Treatment of Pre-skin Cancer   33
Joyce B. Farah, James Ralston, Nathalie C. Zeitouni, Allan R. Oseroff

4 Treatment as Prevention for Skin Cancer   53
Catherine Maari, Robert Bissonnette

5 Treatment of Skin Cancer   65
Sigrid Karrer, Rolf-Markus Szeimies

6 Treatment of Human Papilloma Virus   77
Ida Marie Stender

7 Other Dermatologic Indications for ALA-PDT   89
Erin M. Welch, Kristen M. Kelly

8 Skin Rejuvenation   101
Jaggi Rao, Mitchel P. Goldman, Michael H. Gold

Index   115

Series Foreword
Procedures in Cosmetic Dermatology

While dermatologists have been procedurally inclined since the beginning of the specialty, particularly rapid change has occurred in the past quarter century. The advent of frozen section technique and the golden age of Mohs skin cancer surgery has led to the formal incorporation of surgery within the dermatology curriculum. More recently technological breakthroughs in minimally invasive procedural dermatology have offered an aging population new options for improving the appearance of damaged skin.

Procedures for rejuvenating the skin and adjacent regions are actively sought by our patients. Significantly, dermatologists have pioneered devices, technologies and medications, which have continued to evolve at a startling pace. Numerous major advances, including virtually all cutaneous lasers and light-source based procedures, botulinum exotoxin, soft-tissue augmentation, dilute anesthesia liposuction, leg vein treatments, chemical peels, and hair transplants, have been invented, or developed and enhanced by dermatologists. Dermatologists understand procedures, and we have special insight into the structure, function, and working of skin. Cosmetic dermatologists have made rejuvenation accessible to risk-averse patients by emphasizing safety and reducing operative trauma. No specialty is better positioned than dermatology to lead the field of cutaneous surgery while meeting patient needs.

As dermatology grows as a specialty, an ever-increasing proportion of dermatologists will become proficient in the delivery of different procedures. Not all dermatologists will perform all procedures, and some will perform very few, but even the less procedurally directed amongst us must be well-versed in the details to be able to guide and educate our patients. Whether you are a skilled dermatologic surgeon interested in further expanding your surgical repertoire, a complete surgical novice wishing to learn a few simple procedures, or somewhere in between, this book and this series is for you.

The volume you are holding is one of a series entitled "Procedures in Cosmetic Dermatology." The purpose of each book is to serve as a practical primer on a major topic area in procedural dermatology.

If you want make sure you find the right book for your needs, you may wish to know what this book is and what it is not. It is not a comprehensive text grounded in theoretical underpinnings. It is not exhaustively referenced. It is not designed to be a completely unbiased review of the world's literature on the subject. At the same time, it is not an overview of cosmetic procedures that describes these in generalities without providing enough specific information to actually permit someone to perform the procedures. And importantly, it is not so heavy that it can serve as a doorstop or a shelf filler.

What this book and this series offer is a step-by-step, practical guide to performing cutaneous surgical procedures. Each volume in the series has been edited by a known authority in that subfield. Each editor has recruited other equally practical-minded, technically skilled, hands-on clinicians to write the constituent chapters. Most chapters have two authors to ensure that different approaches and a broad range of opinions are incorporated. On the other hand, the two authors and the editors also collectively provide a consistency of tone. A uniform template has been used within each chapter so that the reader will be easily able to navigate all the books in the series. Within every chapter, the authors succinctly tell it like they do it. The emphasis is on therapeutic technique; treatment methods are discussed with an eye to appropriate indications, adverse events, and unusual cases. Finally, this book is short and can be read in its entirety on a long plane ride. We believe that brevity paradoxically results in greater information transfer because cover-to-cover mastery is practicable.

We hope you enjoy this book and the rest of the books in the series and that you benefit from the many hours of clinical wisdom that have been distilled to produce it. Please keep it nearby, where you can reach for it when you need it.

Jeffrey S. Dover MD FRCPC and Murad Alam MD

To the women in my life

My grandmothers, Bertha and Lillian
My mother, Nina
My daughters, Sophie and Isabel
And especially to my wife, Tania

For their never-ending encouragement, patience, support, love, and friendship

To my father, Mark
A great teacher and role model

To my mentor, Kenneth A. Arndt for his generosity, kindness, sense of humor, joie de vivre, and above all else curiosity and enthusiasm

At Elsevier, Sue Hodgson who conceptualized the series and brought it to reality

and

Martin Mellor for polite, persistent, and dogged determination.

Jeffrey S. Dover

The professionalism of the dedicated editorial staff at Elsevier has made this ambitious project possible. Guided by the creative vision of Sue Hodgson, Martin Mellor and Shuet-Kei Cheung have attended to the myriad tasks required to produce a state-of-the-art resource. In this, they have been ably supported by the graphics team, which has maintained production quality while ensuring portability. We are also deeply grateful to the volume editors, who have generously found time in their schedules, cheerfully accepted our guidelines, and recruited the most knowledgeable chapter authors. Finally, we thank the chapter contributors, without whose work there would be no books at all. Whatever successes are herein are due to the efforts of the above, and of my teachers, Kenneth Arndt, Jeffrey Dover, Michael Kaminer, Leonard Goldberg, and David Bickers, and of my parents, Rahat and Rehana Alam.

Murad Alam

Preface

Photodynamic Therapy (PDT) dates from 1400 BC, when a variety of botanical products were used to improve phototherapy. PDT was first used as a treatment for skin cancer 100 years ago in 1905 by Drs. Von Tappeiner and Jodblauer. Over this past century, physicians have been experimenting with a variety of compounds that can preferentially concentrate in various internal and external tumors or benign structures such as hair follicles and sebaceous glands and be activated by light to provide localized destruction. Many such compounds have been tested and are effective in treating a variety of lesions. However, prolonged photosensitivity and the lack of adequate treatment specificity has hampered the widespread acceptance of PDT as a viable treatment modality.

To overcome the adverse effects of systemically administered photosensitizing agents, topical agents have been studied. In 1999, 5-aminolevulinic acid (5-ALA) (Levulan, Dusa Pharmaceuticals) was the first topical photosensitizing agent to receive approval by the US Food and Drug Administration, in this case for the treatment of actinic keratosis. However, researchers worldwide realized that 5-ALA could be used to treat a wide variety of dermatologic conditions. It is therefore fitting that a textbook be compiled to summarize world-wide research on novel PDT strategies. In this text, some of the leading medical research scientists from the United States, Japan, Canada, Germany and Denmark present their published research and speculate regarding future applications of PDT. Our purpose is to present the reader with an up-to-date account on the use of this modality for the treatment of a wide variety of cutaneous disorders.

The future of PDT looks bright. This text provides evidence that PDT has left the laboratory setting and is appropriately becoming part of our everyday practices. In addition to therapeutic efficacy in treating cutaneous disease, cosmetic improvements are seen in a variety of cutaneous concerns including photorejuvenation and acne vulgaris. The introduction of short-contact, full face/broad area PDT treatment makes this therapy a particularly practical alternative: it is safe, efficacious, and relatively pain-free, without significant adverse effects, and commercially available for widespread use. Clinicians should be ready for this new therapeutic approach, which may alter how dermatologists treat photodamage, sebaceous hyperplasia, acne vulgaris, and a variety of other conditions at the juncture between medical dermatology and cosmetic dermatologic surgery.

Mitchel P. Goldman MD

List of Contributors

Robert Bissonnette MD FRCPC
Dermatologist, Innovaderm Research,
Montreal, QC, Canada

Joyce B. Farah MD
Resident and Assistant Clinical Instructor,
Department of Dermatology, Roswell Park
Cancer Institute, Buffalo, NY, USA

Michael H. Gold MD
Consultant Dermatologist, Gold Skin
Care Centre, Nashville, TN, USA

Mitchel P. Goldman MD
Associate Clinical Professor of
Dermatology/Medicine, University of
California, San Diego; Medical Director,
La Jolla SpaMD, La Jolla, CA, USA

Yoshiyasu Itoh MD PhD
Director, Daikanyama Clinic of
Dermatology and Plastic Surgery,
Tokyo, Japan

Sigrid Karrer MD PhD
Assistant Professor, Department of
Dermatology, Regensburg University
Hospital, Germany

Kristen M. Kelly MD
Associate Clinical Professor of
Dermatology, Beckman Laser Institute
and Medical Clinic, University of
California, Irvine, CA, USA

Catherine Maari MD FRCPC
Clinical Instructor, Department of
Dermatology, University of Montreal
Hospital Center, Montreal; Innovaderm
Research, Montreal, QC, Canada

Allan R. Oseroff MD PhD
Professor and Chair of Dermatology,
Roswell Park Cancer Institute, Buffalo,
NY, USA

James Ralston MD
Resident and Assistant Clinical Instructor,
Department of Dermatology, Roswell
Park Cancer Institute, Buffalo, NY, USA

Jaggi Rao MD FRCPC
Associate Clinical Professor of Medicine,
Division of Dermatology and Cutaneous
Sciences, University of Alberta,
Edmonton, Alberta, Canada

Ida Marie Stender MD PhD
Private Practice, Charlottenlund
Dermatology Clinic, Copenhagen,
Denmark

Rolf-Markus Szeimies MD PhD
Associate Professor, Department of
Dermatology, Regensburg University
Hospital, Germany

Erin M. Welch MD
Dermatology Resident Physician,
Department of Dermatology, University of
California-Irvine, Orange, CA, USA

Nathalie C. Zeitouni MDCM
FRCPC
Chief of Dermatologic Surgery; Associate
Professor of Clinical Dermatology;
Director of Dermatologic Surgery Training,
Roswell Park Cancer Institute, State
University of New York, Buffalo, NY, USA

Brian D. Zelickson MD
Assistant Professor, Department of
Dermatology, University of Minnesota,
Minneapolis, MN, USA

1

Mechanism of Action of Topical Aminolevulinic Acid

Brian D. Zelickson

Introduction

Mechanism of action

In photodynamic therapy (PDT), a chemical reaction activated by light energy is used to selectively destroy tissue. The reaction requires a photosensitive chemical (photosensitizer) in the target tissue and a light source that emits wavelengths absorbed by the chemical. The reaction produces singlet oxygen ($^1O_2$) and other free radicals that are cytotoxic (see Box 1.1). Singlet oxygen's radius of cytotoxic action is $> 0.02\,\mu m$ and its lifetime in biological systems is $< 0.04\,\mu s$. PDT has many applications in medicine because the photosensitizer accumulates preferentially in abnormal tissue, thus localizing the cytotoxic effects of the reaction products. Temporary cutaneous photosensitivity is the most frequent adverse effect of PDT.

Evolution of PDT

Light-based therapy is not new. The use of exogenous photosensitizers to improve the efficacy of phototherapy was described in the Atharva Veda, a sacred Indian book dating back to 1400 BC. By 1900 Raab had described the phototoxic effects of natural dyes. Three years later, Jesionek and Tappeiner used the dye eosin and light to successfully treat skin cancer. In the early 1960s, Lipson and Schwartz of the Mayo Clinic injected hematoporphyrins—a fluorescent mixture of porphyrins—into a patient undergoing surgery and noted fluorescence in neoplastic tissue, demonstrating the photosensitizer's localization in tumors.

Photofrin

From the hematoporphyrin studies came porfimer sodium (Photofrin, QLT Phototherapeutics Inc., Vancouver, BC, Canada), a purified mixture of porphyrins and the first photosensitizer for PDT to obtain governmental clearance for human use. When administered intravenously, porfimer sodium is selectively retained in tumors as compared to normal tissue. This property made it possible to treat tumors that could be illuminated, such as those in the skin and the gastrointestinal, genitourinary, and pulmonary tracts. Porfimer sodium's main drawback is cutaneous photosensitivity; patients must avoid sun exposure for weeks after treatment.

Levulan and Metvix

To overcome the limitations of systemically administered photosensitizers, investigators began to study photosensitizing agents that could be topically applied. Research resulted in the 1999 US Food and Drug Administration (FDA) clearance of Levulan Kerastick (5-aminolevulinic acid HCl, Dusa Pharmaceuticals, Inc.) for the treatment of multiple actinic keratoses (AKs) on the scalp and head and the 2001 European approval of Metvix (methylaminolevulinate, PhotoCure ASA) PDT for the treatment of AK and basal cell carcinoma (BCC). Figure 1.1 shows the structures of both products.

Production of cytotoxic singlet oxygen and other free radicals in target tissue

$$\text{Photosensitive chemical} + \text{light} \longrightarrow {}^1O_2 + \text{free radicals}$$

Box 1.1 Production of cytotoxic singlet oxygen and other free radicals in target tissue

For cutaneous applications, the photosensitizer is usually produced endogenously by first applying the photosensitizing agent to the skin. For example, 5-aminolevulinic acid (ALA) can act as a photosensitizing agent. Though not photosensitive, ALA applied to the skin penetrates into underlying tissue, where it is converted to protoporphyrin IX (PpIX), a photosensitive compound. When ALA is applied to tumors of epidermal origin such as BCCs and squamous cell carcinomas (SCCs), strong fluorescence due to PpIX is observed.

In PDT, a source that emits light at wavelengths within the absorption spectrum of the photosensitizer must be available. The time between photo-sensitizer administration and light application should be within practical limits (e.g. several hours). The longer the wavelength, the deeper the light penetrates tissue. Light at 630 nm penetrates up to 5 mm while 700–800 nm light may reach up to 2 cm. Longer wavelengths lack sufficient energy to activate a useful photochemical reaction.

A variety of photosensitive chemicals and light sources have been used in PDT. This chapter focuses on the uses of topically applied ALA and methylaminolevulinate (MALA), the light sources used to activate the endogenously produced porphyrins, and the cosmetic/dermatologic applications of PDT.

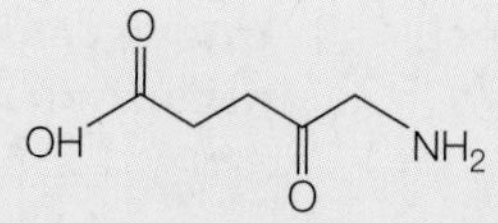

(a) 5-Aminolevulinic acid HCL (Levulan® Kerastick®, Dusa Pharmaceuticals, Inc.)

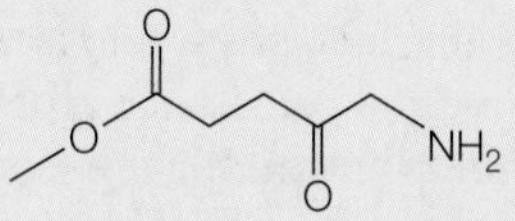

(b) Methylaminolevulinate (Metvix®, PhotoCure ASA)

Fig. 1.1 Structures of Levulan and Metvix

Photosensitizers

An ideal photosensitizer is: (1) minimally toxic, (2) taken up more quickly by abnormal (target) tissue than by normal tissue, (3) cleared rapidly from normal tissue, (4) activated at wavelengths that penetrate the target tissue, and (5) capable of producing large amounts of cytotoxic product. Photosensitizers in use or under investigation for cutaneous indications are shown in Table 1.1.

How photosensitizers kill cells

Photosensitizers useful in PDT are taken up by both normal and rapidly dividing (malignant) cells, but cleared less rapidly from neoplastic cells. This difference in clearance rate may be due to the greater number and permeability of blood vessels and slower lymphatic drainage in rapidly dividing

Photosensitizers and potential indications for cutaneous malignancies			
Sensitizer	**Trade name**	**Potential indications**	**Activation wavelength**
Photofrin			
BPD-MA	Verteporfin	BCC	689 nm
ALA	Levulan	BCC	635 nm
MALA	Metvix	BCC	635 nm
SnET2	Purlytin	BCC, cutaneous metastatic breast cancer	664 nm
HPPH	Photochlor	BCC	665 nm
Phthalocyanine-4	Pc 4	Cutaneous/subcutaneous lesions from diverse solid tumor groups	670 nm

BPD-MA = benzoporphyrin derivative monoacid ring A, ALA = 5-aminolevulinic acid, MALA = methylaminolevulinate, SnET2 = tin etiopurpurin dichloride, HPPH = 2-[1-hexyloxyethyl]-2-devinyl pyropheophorbide-a.
Adapted with permission of Dolmans DE, Fukumura D, Jain RK 2003 Photodynamic therapy for cancer. Nature Review of Cancer 3:380–387)

Table 1.1 Photosensitizers and potential indications for cutaneous malignancies

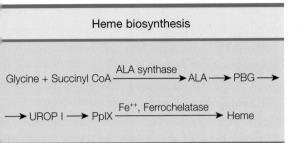

Box 1.2 Heme biosynthesis

neoplastic cells. Photosensitizers are believed to localize in blood vessels, lysosomes, mitochondria, plasma membranes, and nuclei of tumor cells. PDT kills tumor cells by: (1) direct destruction by singlet oxygen, (2) damage to blood vessels, and (3) activation of an immune response.

Porphyrins

Porphyrin-based photosensitizers, especially porfimer sodium, have been used to treat cancers of the bladder, lung, esophagus, stomach, skin, and cervix by PDT. Porphyrins absorb maximally at the Soret band (360–400 nm) and have four smaller peaks of between 500 and 635 nm. Cutaneous applications of porphyrin sensitizers are limited because clearance of porphyrins is slow, leading to cutaneous photosensitivity for 4–6 weeks. A major advantage of topically applied ALA is that cutaneous photosensitivity is limited to the treated area and lasts only a few days.

Nonporphyrins

Other photosensitizers under investigation include benzoporphyrin derivative (used to treat BCC), SnET2 (used to treat BCC, cutaneous metastatic breast cancer, Kaposi's sarcoma, prostate cancer), chorin derivatives (used to treat BCC), and phthalocyanine-4 (used to treat cutaneous and subcutaneous lesions of many solid tumors).

Topical ALA and MALA

A natural precursor to photosensitive PpIX, ALA is widely used in PDT of cutaneous disorders. The formation of ALA from glycine and succinyl CoA in tissue (in the presence of ALA synthase) is the first and rate-limiting step in heme biosynthesis (Box 1.2). Two molecules of ALA condense enzymatically to form porphobilinogen (PBG), then four PBG molecules are converted to uroporphyrinogen I (UROP I). This leads to the formation of PpIX, to which iron is added in the presence of ferrochelatase to form heme.

Biosynthesis of heme

In the absence of exogenous ALA, the concentration of free heme controls the amount of ALA produced in tissue by feedback inhibition of ALA synthase. When a large amount of ALA is applied to the skin and absorbed by rapidly dividing (abnormal) cells, PpIX concentration increases more rapidly than it can be converted to heme by the available ferrochelatase, leading to a temporary build-up of PpIX. The preferential accumulation of PpIX in certain types of cells (by mechanisms not fully understood) is the basis for the clinical use of ALA in PDT.

Penetration of ALA into skin

The effectiveness of photosensitizing agent depends partly on how deeply and how selectively the agent penetrates the skin. Penetration efficiency of ALA is influenced by the skin thickness and ALA penetrates skin of benign abnormalities (e.g. AKs, sun damage, abrasions, inflammation, psoriasis) more readily than it does normal skin. The generally thicker skin of native Americans and oriental people is less permeable to ALA than the thin skin of Europeans. ALA penetrates heavily freckled skin in an irregularly dotted pattern as shown by observing PpIX fluorescence after ALA application. Superficial BCC and SCC produce abnormal keratin, which is more easily penetrated by ALA than nearby normal skin, suggesting that ALA can be liberally applied on and around the lesion unless the patient has unusually thin or sun-damaged skin.

Treatment experience

When ALA has penetrated deeply enough and has been converted into PpIX, the patient is ready for light treatment. Less than 1 min after exposure to light, most patients report a burning, tingling, or itching that peaks in a few minutes and subsides to the level of a 'mild sunburn' in the treated area. The sensation disappears within 24 h but the treated area may be tender for a few days.

Adverse effects

When treatment is completed, the treated area may be slightly edematous and erythematous. In heavily freckled patients, a histamine-like reaction may occur, with erythema extending up to 10 cm outside the treated lesion. Some patients may develop superficial erosions with weeping and crusting. Patients should be instructed to avoid sun exposure for 24–48 h due to temporary cutaneous photo-toxicity associated with treatment.

Rate of penetration

The rate that PpIX accumulates and is distributed in cutaneous tumors depends on the type of lesion. It has been estimated the ALA requires 3–15 h to penetrate 2.5–3.0 mm into various types of tissue, however it works into AKs in as little as 60 min. Physicians can verify that ALA has entered tissue and become PpIX by observing fluorescence under ultraviolet light (Wood's lamp). With prolonged exposure to light (more than 13 h), ALA-treated lesions become irritated, edematous, and erythematous.

Because ALA is hydrophilic and does not readily penetrate the stratum corneum, a large amount must be applied to skin to assure sufficient absorption for PDT. This drawback stimulated the development of lipophilic esters of ALA (e.g. MALA) to promote more rapid absorption.

Light sources

To be useful in PDT, a light source must emit wavelengths in the absorption spectrum of the photosensitizer. Absorption peaks for porphyrins are at 410 (maximum), 505, 540, 580, and 630 nm. The amount of photoactivation depends on the amount of absorbable light that reaches the photosensitizer in the target tissue. Long wavelengths penetrate more deeply into tissue, but this advantage is limited by how strongly the photosensitizer absorbs light at these long wavelengths. For example, 630 nm light penetrates more deeply into tissue than 410 nm light, but absorption by the porphyrin photosensitizer is much stronger at 410 nm than at 635 nm. In this case, the appropriate wavelength would depend on the depth of the target tumor. If absorption is low, time of exposure to light may be extended or the amount of energy may be increased to achieve photoactivation. Treatment with visible light is accompanied by pain, which can be lessened

by using filters to remove short-wavelength light or by reducing the rate or time of light exposure.

Nonlasers

Lasers and nonlasers have been used with success in PDT for dermatologic conditions. Visible light sources such as halogen, xenon, and fluorescent lamps—even slide projectors—are less expensive and more effective than lasers in treating large lesions or lesions in which depth of penetration is unimportant (e.g. AKs). Nonlaser light sources also do not require the use of safety glasses. In addition, irradiation with multiple wavelengths, as with broadband visible light, can improve efficacy. For example, 630–675 nm light is frequently used in lasers to activate PpIX, but a source that also provides 675 nm light also activates photoprotoporphyrin, a photoproduct of PpIX. The result is greater therapeutic benefit. Dosimetry with visible light, however, may be less accurate than with a laser and stray infrared light from the broadband source may heat the skin, causing pain.

Two blue light sources—the BLU-U PDT Illuminator (Dusa Pharmaceuticals) for the treatment of AK lesions and the ClearLight System (Lumenis) for the treatment of moderate inflammatory acne—have been cleared by the FDA. Intense pulsed light (IPL) at 590–1200 nm has been used for simultaneous skin rejuvenation and removal of AK lesions.

Lasers

With lasers, users can more easily target specific areas, minimize exposure times, and select wavelengths. Pulsed gold vapor, continuous-wave argon pumped dye, copper vapor, KTP and pulsed-dye lasers have been used in dermatologic PDT.

Alternative light dosing

Currently there have been several reports of using high-energy, very short pulsed exposures of light (pulsed-dye lasers, ms pulsed-KTP lasers and IPLs) to activate PpIX after topically applied ALA. Figure 1.2 and Table 1.2 show the relative PpIX activation doses of various lasers and light sources. These studies have shown significant clearance of AK and actinic cheilitis as well as significant improvement in the fine lines, dyspigmentation and

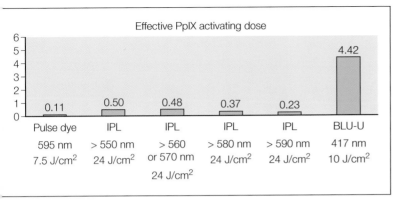

Fig. 1.2 Effective PpIX-activating dose

Effective PpIX-activating doses, updated for various IPL filter settings			
	Dose (J/cm²)	PAE coefficient	Effective dose (J/cm²)	Dose to equal pulsed dye (J/cm²)
Pulsed dye	7.5	0.0150	0.11	7.5
IPL – 550 nm	24	0.0207	0.50	5.4
IPL – 560 or 570 nm	24	0.0198	0.48	5.7
IPL – 580 nm	24	0.0152	0.37	7.4
IPL – 590 nm	24	0.0095	0.23	11.9
BLU-U	10	0.4425	4.42	0.3

Courtesy of DUSA Pharmeceuticals

Table 1.2 Effective PpIX-activating doses, updated for various IPL filter settings

erythema associated with photodamage (Fig. 1.3). The advantage of using these devices is that the treatment is relatively fast and these devices can, unlike ALA-PDT alone, directly clear vessels and pigmentation.

Other investigators have shown that very low dose chemiluminescent light patches (each patch emits 431–515 nm wavelengths of light for a total of 55.6 mJ/cm² over 20 min) over a long exposure time (45–60 min) can produce significant clearing in AK and inflammatory acne. Local treatment effect using topical ALA with a low energy light source shows an early inflammatory response with long-term clearing of the AK (Fig. 1.4). The main potential benefit of this procedure is that these light sources are very inexpensive, disposable and may be perfect for home use.

Both of these types of activations, although of utility in the clinical setting, have not been shown to produce a PDT reaction in in vitro studies. Osoroff has performed in vitro phototoxicity assays using tumor cell cultures incubated with ALA and exposed to a pulsed-dye laser using 595 nm, 10 spot size and 6 ms pulse duration (5 J/cm²) pulsing ten times (50 J/cm²) as well as the low energy light patch described earlier. These in vitro experiments resulted in no significant cell killing.

This gives rise to the question of how this light activation works. It appears to be different from the way most PDT works. There may be enough activation of PpIX in order to stimulate a host immune response against the surrounding structures, or there may be other unexplained mechanisms. One simple explanation is that since most of the areas studied are on the face, which cannot be adequately protected from light exposure, these short pulsed and low-level long pulsed exposures do not activate much of the PpIX and the reaction mostly occurs over the next several days by incidental exposure to light. However, Ross has shown very good PpIX activation on sun protected skin after IPL exposure (Fig. 1.5).

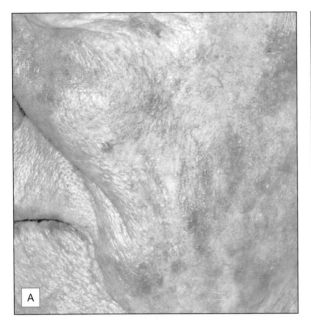

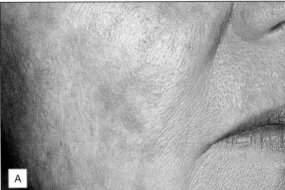

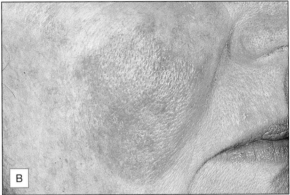

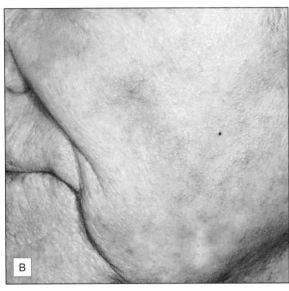

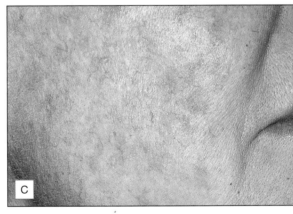

Fig. 1.3 Severe photodamage pre-treatment (**A**) and 3 months after treatment (**B**) with topical ALA (60-minute incubation) and PDL exposure with 595 nm, 6 ms pulse duration, 10 mm spot size

Fig. 1.4 (**A**) pre-treatment showing diffuse AK. (**B**) 1 week follow up after 45-minute ALA incubation and 45-minute exposure using a topical light patch showing erythema and urtication. (**C**) 3-month follow up showing resolution of keratosis

Expected benefits

Clinical benefits of PDT in treating AKs and non-melanoma cutaneous malignancies are summarized in Table 1.3. PDT also shows promise in photorejuvenation, mild to moderate acne, nevus sebaceous of Jadassohn, and sebaceous hyperplasia.

Overview of Treatment Strategy

The following topics will be reviewed in later chapters: treatment approach, major determinants, and patient interviews.

Condition	Light dose (J/cm^2)		CR rate (%)		Follow-up time		Adverse effects
	L	NL	L	NL	L	NL	
AKs	10–150	2–300	91–100	64–100	2 months	1–20 months	Localized pain during light treatment, erythema, edema
BCC	60–250	18–300	50–100	86–97	1–17 months	1–20 months	Localized pain during light treatment, erythema, edema, crusting
Bowen's disease	60–250	62.5–300	89–100	30–98	1–18 months	2–20 months	Localized pain during light treatment, erythema, edema, urticaria, blistering, eschar, hypo-, hyperpigmentation
SCC	60–80	30–540	84	40–100	36 months	3–6 months	Localized pain during treatment, inflammation, necrosis, crusting

CR = complete response (no visible evidence of tumor), L = laser, NL = nonlaser

Table 1.3 Benefits and adverse effects of laser and nonlaser PDT of premalignant and nonmelanoma skin cancers

Treatment techniques

In dermatology, the most extensively studied photo-sensitizing agents for PDT are ALA and MALA. ALA as Levulan Kerastick is currently FDA cleared for the treatment of AKs on the scalp and head and MALA as Metvix is approved in Europe for the treatment of AK and BCC.

Aminolevulinic Acid

Actinic keratoses

Usually caused by sun exposure, AKs occur primarily on the scalp and face of people aged 40 years and older. The goal in removing AKs is to prevent the development of SCC. Metastatic SCC causes 60% of deaths due to nonmelanoma skin cancer.

Conventional treatment

AKs are traditionally removed by cryotherapy (for few lesions), curettage, and 5-fluorouracil (5-FU) for many lesions. The choice of technique depends on the number of lesions, compliance, and tolerance. These modalities, though efficacious, may also cause pain, prolonged erythema, scarring, crusting, hypopigmentation, and hyperpigmentation. Topical

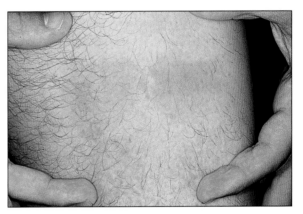

Fig. 1.5 Image taken of the upper thigh after a 24-hour ALA incubation and treatment with the violet hp (Lux V) (Palomar medi lux) using 9 J/cm^2. Note erythema and urtication confined to treated area. (Photograph courtesy of Dr Vic Ross)

imiquimod and diclofenac sodium have become available, but imiquimod can cause crusting and diclofenac may not be as effective as 5-FU.

Advantages of PDT

ALA-PDT has the advantage of selective uptake by AK lesions and abnormal cells of lesions not yet visible. AK lesions are superficial, so depth of penetration by ALA is not as important as in nodular

BCC tumors. Complete response (CR, no visible evidence of tumor) using ALA and a halogen lamp (580–740 nm) at a low dose (20 J/cm^2) have been obtained for diffuse, palpable lesions on the scalp. Although the treatment is painful, remission can be durable.

PDT treatment

Broadband green light, red light, blue light, and laser light (585 nm, 595 nm, and 630 nm) have been used to activate PpIX. Responses are higher with nonhypertrophic than with hypertrophic lesions. Lesions on the hands and arms have been treated with PDT, but with less success than with facial lesions. Erythema, edema, burning, and stinging usually accompany treatment, but most patients do not require anesthesia. Light treatment with PDL (585 nm) or cryogen spray cooling with 595 nm PDL activation may result in less pain than broadband light irradiation.

In the phase III trials of Levulan with blue light (417 nm, BLU-U Blue Light Photodynamic Therapy Illuminator, Dusa Pharmaceuticals, Inc.), 83% of 243 patients with nonhypertrophic AKs had a CR after 2 months. Cosmetic results were good to excellent in more than 90% of lesions. In four trial patients (32 lesions in total) followed for 4 years after treatment, 69% of lesions remained clear, 9% recurred, and 22% were classified as 'uncertain.'

In the initial studies of ALA-PDT in the treatment of AKs, ALA was in contact with skin under occlusive dressing for 3–20 hours before light treatment. The Levulan package insert recommends 14–18 hours' application time (see Chapter 3).

Basal cell carcinoma
Conventional treatment

The most common cutaneous malignant disease, BCC may be treated by surgical excision, Mohs' surgery, cryosurgery, radiation therapy, curettage, and electrodesiccation. ALA-PDT is an option for patients (1) hesitant to undergo surgery due to poor health, (2) who have recently undergone radiation therapy, or (3) with many superficial tumors.

PDT treatment

For superficial BCC, complete response rates are 79–100% compared to 10–70% for nodular BCC,

the difference likely due to limited penetration of ALA into deeper layers of the nodular tumor. Response rates for nodular BCC tumors have been improved by repeated treatment sessions using dimethyl sulfoxide (DMSO), ethylenediamine tetraacetic acid (EDTA), or desferrioxamine to enhance ALA penetration, or allowing ALA to remain in contact with tumor for more than 6 h.

Recurrence rates are lowest with superficial BCC tumors < 2 mm thick. One group obtained 9% recurrence of BCC after 45 months, but earlier reports suggest recurrence rates up to 50%. The wide range of outcomes may be related to the different treatment conditions used by different investigators.

Lasers and broadband lamps are equally effective in activating PpIX for BCC except that high light doses may be more difficult to deliver with a lamp. Adverse effects are similar to those of AK—localized pain during treatment, erythema, edema, and crusting (see Chapter 5).

Bowen's disease
Conventional treatment

Bowen's disease, or SCC in situ, is currently treated by cryotherapy, topical 5-FU, curettage, electrocautery, radiotherapy, or surgical excision. Comparison studies show that ALA-PDT is more effective and has fewer side effects than either cryotherapy or topical 5-FU. Unlike cryotherapy, ALA-PDT is not associated with infection, ulceration, or scar formation. PDT is also less painful than cryotherapy. Topical 5-FU treatment may be accompanied by eczematous reactions, ulceration, and erosion, which have not been reported with PDT.

PDT treatment

ALA-PDT is of potential utility for large patches (40–80 mm diameter) of Bowen's disease not amenable to other modalities. ALA penetration depth is not critical because Bowen's tumors are intraepidermal, but treatment should be approached with caution since occult invasive foci less amenable to ALA-PDT may exist within a superficial-appearing lesion. For Bowen's disease, ALA is typically in contact with skin for 4–8 h under occlusion before light treatment. Lasers and broadband light are both effective, although response rates are higher with red light (615–645 nm) than with green light (525–555 nm). Response rates with one to two treatment sessions are 89–100% and recurrence rates are 10% or less for up to 18 months.

Adverse effects include localized pain during light treatment, erythema, edema, urticaria, blistering, eschar formation, hypopigmentation, and hyperpigmentation. All resolve without intervention.

Squamous cell carcinoma
Conventional treatment

SCC is the second most common type of skin cancer. Conventional treatment includes excision or destruction depending upon the clinical situation. If standard methods are contraindicated, PDT may be a treatment option, however the recurrence rates can be high and the risk for catastrophic outcomes such as metastasis cannot be completely eliminated.

PDT treatment

Complete response rates with ALA-PDT vary from 40% to 100% with one or more treatment sessions. Repetitive ALA-PDT for superficial nonmelanoma skin cancers has showed histological CR rates of 83% for superficial SCC and 33% for nodular SCC in patients followed for 24–36 months after treatment. ALA has been applied for 6–8 h and lesions treated with 630 nm light from a dye laser. Comparable results with fewer patients and broadband visible light have been reported (see Chapter 5).

Sebaceous disorders
Acne

Conventional treatment for acne consists of topical formulations, oral antibiotics, and isotretinoin. Topical formulations may irritate the skin, *Propionibacterium acnes* may resist oral antibiotics, and isotretinoin is teratogenic, expensive, and unavailable in some countries.

Researchers have begun to develop PDT parameters to treat acne because:

- sun exposure improves acne lesions
- *P. acnes* produces porphyrins that absorb at 415 nm
- irradiating *P. acnes* with blue light activates bacterial porphyrins, generates singlet oxygen, and destroys bacteria
- ALA is absorbed by pilosebaceous glands and converted to PpIX
- irradiation with blue and red light alone or combined improves mild to moderate acne.

In early studies, ALA and red light improved acne lesions but dosimetry parameters produced pain during treatment, erythema, exfoliation, and hyperpigmentation that caused patients to postpone treatments. Seborrhea often returned and more acne lesions appeared within 6 months.

Pain during treatment and other adverse effects were reduced when either of two blue light sources (BLU-U with ALA and ClearLight [Lumenis] alone) were used in patients with mild to moderate acne. Both sources are FDA approved for the treatment of moderate inflammatory acne.

Goldman and Boyce treated 22 patients with moderate to severe acne. Patients received either ALA followed by BLU-U irradiation or BLU-U alone once a week for 2 weeks. Acne severity improved 2 weeks later (32% vs. 25%), papule counts decreased 68% vs. 40%, and pustule counts decreased 61% vs. 65% in ALA-BLU-U treatment groups and BLU-U alone groups, respectively. Using the Clearlight source alone, another group reduced acne lesions 64% in patients treated twice weekly for 5 weeks. A third group reported comparable results with the Clearlight system in patients with papulo-pustular acne treated according to three 4-week protocols.

Either the BLU-U or Clearlight protocols offer a treatment alternative to acne patients wishing to avoid the disadvantages of conventional treatments. A complete discussion is found in Chapter 2.

Nevus sebaceous of Jadassohn

In a case report, a lesion of nevus sebaceous of Jadassohn (NSJ) was flattened and reduced in size with 13 ALA-PDT treatment sessions spaced 4–8 weeks apart. No serious adverse effects were reported and the lesion had not returned for 16 months after the final treatment. A tunable dye laser (630 nm) was used at $100\,J/cm^2$ total dose.

Sebaceous hyperplasia

Treatment modalities for sebaceous hyperplasia (SH) include cryotherapy, cauterization, oral isotretinoin, ablative laser vaporization, and surgical excision. These may be painful, require repeated treatment sessions, and cause scarring.

ALA-PDT offers a treatment option with a good cosmetic outcome. In a 61-year-old man, topically applied ALA (4 h) and visible light irradiation with a red glass filter in once-weekly treatment sessions for 3 weeks reduced the size of large SH lesions and nearly resolved small lesions. Edema and hyperpigmentation resolved within 10 days after the last treatment. In a 10-patient study by Alster, 1-hour ALA application followed by irradiation with a 595 nm PDL cleared the papules of all patients in one to two treatment sessions with mild adverse effects.

Photorejuvenation

Investigators have begun to explore ALA-PDT as a noninvasive, no-downtime option in photorejuvenation.

The IPL has been used to treat photodamaged skin for improvement in irregular pigmentation, skin coarseness, and telangiectasias. The procedure does not clear AKs, which would have to be removed as a separate procedure (see Chapter 8).

PDT-IPL

To include removal of AKs as part of a single photorejuvenation procedure, Ruiz-Rodriguez et al combined IPL with ALA-PDT in two treatment sessions 1 month apart. In each session, the investigators applied ALA for 4 h and used IPL to clear 33 of 38 AK lesions for at least 3 months in 17 patients. Treatment parameters using an IPL device were the following: a 615 nm cutoff filter and $40 J/cm^2$ with a 4.0 ms double-pulse mode and 40 ms delay time between pulses. Of the 38 AKs, 29 were resolved after the first treatment. The five uncleared AKs were greatly improved.

The procedure was well tolerated, no scars or changes in pigmentation occurred, and erythema and crusting in the AK areas resolved within 1 week. Patients had Fitzpatrick skin types II and III. EMLA was applied to the nonAK area for 2 h before treatment.

The procedure has not been evaluated in patients with diffuse AKs or in its long-term efficacy.

PDT with blue light

ALA-PDT with blue light has also shown encouraging results. In a study of two patients with moderately photodamaged skin, skin elasticity improved and skin thickening was reduced in facial areas in which multiple nonhyperkeratotic AKs had been cleared by ALA-PDT with blue light.

Touma et al used PDT with 1–3-hour ALA application time and blue light $(10 J/cm^2)$ to improve skin quality, fine wrinkling, and sallowness in 18 patients with moderate diffuse facial sun damage and at least four nonhypertrophic AKs. Mottled pigmentation had borderline improvement and coarse wrinkling showed no improvement. Satisfaction was good to excellent in more than 80% of patients. The investigators suggested using microdermabrasion immediately before treatment for more uniform and rapid penetration of ALA and removal of stratum corneum.

Methylaminolevulinate for AK

Metvix, a lipophilic methyl ester of ALA, is approved in Europe for the treatment of AK and BCC. In the USA, the photosensitizing agent has an FDA approvability letter for the treatment of AK, but is not yet cleared for marketing. When MALA is used as a photosensitizing agent in PDT, adverse effects are similar to those of ALA-PDT.

Treatment of AK with MALA-PDT has been studied by two groups. In a 204-patient study, Freeman et al found that two treatments with MALA-PDT (red light, 570–670 nm, $75 J/cm^2$) resulted in a 91% CR rate 3 months after treatment compared to 68% for cryotherapy. MALA PDT treatment sessions were 1 week apart and MALA was in contact with treated areas for 3 h before irradiation. Another group reported similar response rates for MALA-PDT in an 80-patient study.

Further Reading

Alster TS, Tanzi EL 2003 Photodynamic therapy with topical aminolevulinic acid and pulsed dye laser irradiation for sebaceous hyperplasia. Journal of Drugs in Dermatology 2:501–504

Dolmans DE, Fukumura D, Jain RK 2003 Photodynamic therapy for cancer. National Review of Cancer 3:380–387

Freeman M, Vinciullo C, Francis D et al 2003 A comparison of photodynamic therapy using topical methyl aminolevulinate (Metvix) with single cycle cryotherapy in patients with actinic keratosis: a prospective, randomized study. Journal of Dermatologic Treatment 14:99–106

Goldman MP, Boyce SM 2003 A single-center study of aminolevulinic acid and 417 nm photodynamic therapy in the treatment of moderate to severe acne vulgaris. Journal of Drugs in Dermatology 2:393–396

Jeffes EW 2002 Levulan: the first approved topical photosensitizer for the treatment of actinic keratosis. Journal of Dermatologic Treatment 13(suppl 1):S19–S23

Kalka K, Merk H, Mukhtar H 2000 Photodynamic therapy in dermatology. Journal of the American Academy of Dermatology 42:389–413

Marcus SL, McIntire WR 2002 Photodynamic therapy systems and applications. Expert Opinion in Emerging Drugs 7:319–331

Piacquadio DJ, Chen DM, Farber HF et al 2004 Photodynamic therapy with aminolevulinic acid topical solution and visible blue light in the treatment of multiple actinic keratoses of the face and scalp: investigator-blinded, phase 3, multicenter trials. Archives of Dermatology 140:41–46

Ruiz-Rodriguez R, Sanz-Sanchez T, Cordoba S 2002 Photodynamic photorejuvenation. Dermatologic Surgery 28:742–744

Sadick NS, Weiss R, Kilmer S et al 2004 Photorejuvenation with intense pulsed light: results of a multi-center study. Journal of Drugs in Dermatology 3:41–49

Taub AF 2004 Photodynamic therapy in dermatology: history and horizons. Journal of Drugs in Dermatology 3(suppl 1):S8–S25

Touma DJ, Gilchrest BA 2003 Topical photodynamic therapy: a new tool in cosmetic dermatology. Seminars in Cutaneous Medical Surgery 22:124–130

Weiss RA, McDaniel DH, Geronemus RG 2003 Review of nonablative photorejuvenation: reversal of the aging effects of the sun and environmental damage using laser and light sources. Seminars in Cutaneous Medical Surgery 22(2):93–106

Treatment of Acne

2

Yoshiyasu Itoh

Introduction

The problem being treated

Acne vulgaris is a common skin disease for adolescent and young adults. Although a small number of acne lesions may be tolerable and easily treated, repeated recalcitrant acne is hard to cure and has a tendency to lead to scarring, causing further distress. Complete freedom from the chronic pimpled condition is very difficult to achieve, although many methods have been introduced. In order to attempt to solve this problem, photodynamic therapy (PDT) aminolevulinic acid (ALA) treatment can be used as a primary regimen. Post-treatment management is necessary to preserve the improvements achieved by PDT-ALA. This chapter provides guidance on how to treat acne with PDT-ALA treatment and how to successfully diminish apparently incurable acne.

Hyperpigmentation after topical ALA-PDT has been observed with very high frequency in Asian patients because of melanogenesis and epidermal exfoliation, which occurs via photodynamic action due to the accumulation of protoporphyrin IX (PpIX) in the epidermis (Figs 2.1, 2.2). More recently, oral administration of ALA has been used for treating acne, and this technique is described later (Figs 2.3, 2.4).

A major cause of acne inflammation is believed to be an increase in perilesional pathogenic bacteria, especially *Propionibacterium acnes (P. acnes)*. Patients undergoing long-term dosage with antibiotics are frequently infected with a number of bacteria, but not always *P. acnes* (Tables 2.1 and 2.2), which may be seen more frequently in more seriously infected patients. However, PDT-ALA treatment is more successful at eradicating *P. acnes* than other bacteria because the available photosensitizers in acne patients

Acne grading by Burton scale	
Grade 0	Total absence of lesions
Grade I	Sub clinical Acne – Few comedons visible only in close examination
Grade II	Comedonal Acne – Comedons with slight inflammation
Grade III	Mild Acne – Inflamed papules with erythema
Grade IV	Moderate Acne – Many inflamed papules and pustules
Grade V	Severe Nodular Acne – Inflamed papules and pustules with several deep modular lesions
Grade VI	Severe Cystic Acne – Many nodular cystic lesions with scarring

Table 2.1 Acne grading by Burton scale

Species of bacteria in 39 serious acne patients (Grades 4–6 on the Burton scale)	
Species of bacteria	**No.**
P. acnes	2
P. acnes + S. epidermis	12
P. acnes + MSSA	3
P. acnes + MRSA	3
P. acnes + S. epidermis + MSSA	1
P. acnes + S. epidermis + MRSA	2
S. epidermis	6
MSSA	1
MRSA	3
MSSA + S. epidermis	2
MRSA + S. epidermis	2
P. acnes + S. epidermis + S. capitis	1
P. acnes + S. epidermis + S. hominis	1

Table 2.2 Species of bacteria in 39 serious acne patients (Grades 4–6 on the Burton scale)

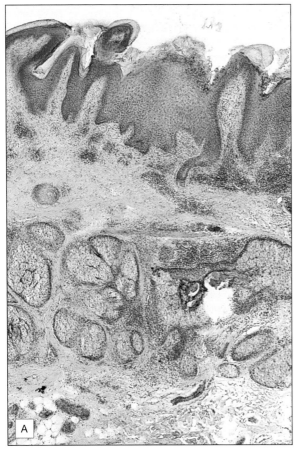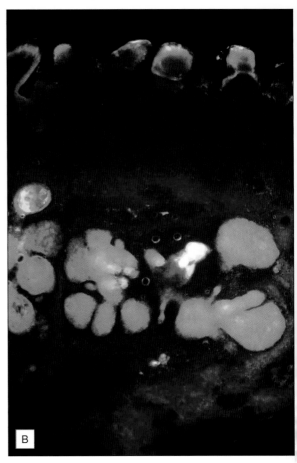

Fig. 2.1 Twelve hours after topical application of 20% ALA ointment, the upper half of the epidermis (**A**) and the whole sebaceous gland (**B**) in sebaceous nevus show fluorescence due to accumulation of PpIX. The eccrine gland does not show fluorescence

Ultraviolet examination

Ultraviolet pictures can easily show the amount of porphyrin as fluorescence and are very useful for judging the bacterial conditions of the patient's skin. If there is no dosing with photosensitizers, the presence of fluorescence means the appearance of endogenous porphyrin (mostly coproporphyrin) produced by *P. acnes*. Healthy controls and most patients undergoing treatment with antibiotics at a low dosage demonstrate fluorescence well (Figs 2.5, 2.6, see page 18). On the other hand, patients with a serious acne condition frequently present less fluorescence, which means that acne lesions are caused by other bacteria but not *P. acnes* (Figs 2.7, 2.8, see page 19). The oral administration of external ALA produces an accumulation of PpIX in the pilosebaceous units and induces more production of coproporphyrin to *P. acnes*. As a result, enhancement of fluorescence is seen (Fig. 2.9, see page 20). On topical application of ALA, fluorescence caused by the accumulation of PpIX in the upper half of the epidermis is seen.

Box 2.1 Ultraviolet examination

infected with *P. acnes* are endogenous coproporphyrin and PpIX associated with external dosage of ALA, while in patients with other bacteria the only operative photosensitizer is PpIX. Before PDT-ALA treatment, it is important to know whether the main bacterium in lesions is *P. acnes*, as eradication of bacteria apart from *P. acnes* may require more PDT procedures. To answer this question, ultraviolet examination is useful (Box 2.1).

Patient selection

A major effect of PDT-ALA treatment of acne is bactericidal. The secondary effect is damage to the sebaceous glands. PDT-ALA treatment can be used for all types of acne and acne in all areas. Moreover, folliculitis, rosacea and seborrhea are also likely to respond to PDT (Fig 2.10, see page 20). Although most acne patients have accompanying seborrhea,

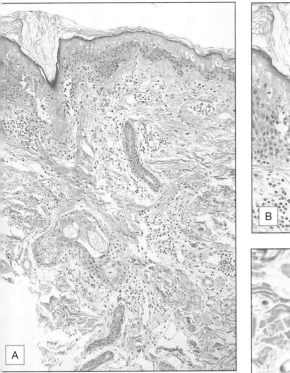

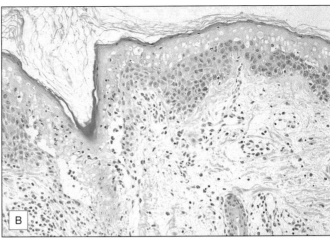

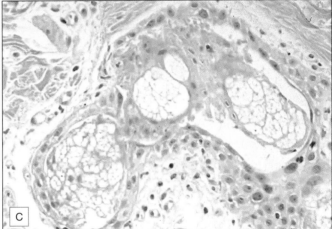

Fig. 2.2 Two days after PDT treatment to the sebaceous nevus in Figure 2.1, the upper half of the epidermis (**A**) and the inner sheath of the hair follicle (**B**) show apoptosis, and the damage to the sebaceous gland (**C**) is seen. The basal pigmentation in the epidermis is observed

patients with dry skin or atopic dermatitis may have a more complicated treatment regimen. Although patients with dry skin can be treated with PDT-ALA treatment, they may need adequate moisturizing skin care as sebaceous glands are destroyed. Generally, sebum secretion is restored 1 month after one session of PDT-ALA treatment. Monthly repeated PDT-ALA treatments can improve seborrhea.

Expected benefits

The results of 96 acne patients treated with orally administered ALA-based PDT are shown. All patients, 30 men and 66 women, were grades 4–6 on the Burton scale (see Table 2.1) and underwent PDT after a 4-week washout period. The average age of the patients was 28 years. As 38 patients were treated on both the face and body, the total numbers of patients treated for facial acne and body acne

were 83 and 51, respectively. Four hours after the oral administration of ALA at 10 mg/kg BW, acne lesions were exposed to polychromatic visible light by a metal halide lamp. All patients underwent between two and four sessions of PDT (one PDT series) and received no other treatments. Each PDT course lasted between 2 and 4 weeks. Based on the photographs before and 3 months after the final PDT treatment, the numbers of papulopustular lesions, but not comedonal lesions, were counted, and the physician's rating assessment of 'worsened', 'unchanged', 'improved', or 'markedly improved' was obtained. All patients were interviewed about adverse effects.

The average reductions in papulopustular lesions before and after PDT-ALA treatments were 12% for facial acne and 18% for body acne, respectively (Figs 2.11–2.13, see pages 21 and 22). The rating assessments for the facial and body acne are summarized

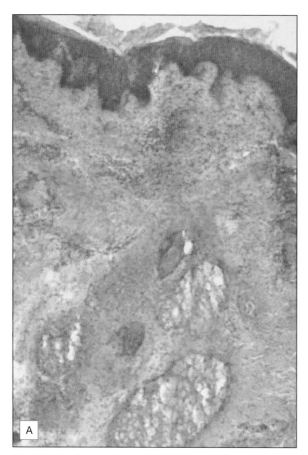
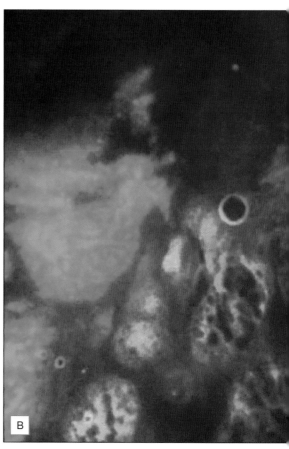

Fig. 2.3 Four hours after oral administration of ALA of 10 mg/kg body weight (BW), fluorescence in the normal skin, due to the accumulation of PpIX, is seen in the pilosebaceous unit but not the epidermis

in Table 2.3. In the rating assessment for facial acne, 0 (0%) were worsened, 7 (8.4%) were unchanged, 26 (31.3%) were improved, and 50 (60.3%) were markedly improved. In the rating assessment for the body acne, the relevant scores were 0 (0%), 4 (7.8%), 16 (31.4%), and 31 (60.8%) patients, respectively.

In this study, almost all patients tolerated the light irradiation, while five patients complained of discomfort, burning, and stinging during the irradiation. Of 96 patients, eight complained of tran-

sient nausea for several hours. Almost all patients developed erythema immediately after PDT treatment. Erythema of the face continued for 1–5 days although most patients recovered within 2 days. Erythema of the body was very mild in most cases and disappeared within 1 day. Five percent of the affected faces showed swelling lasting for 1–5 days. A high degree of erythema and swelling were more often seen in patients with fair skin. Two days after a PDT session, new acne, new pustules and/or hypersecretion of sebum were observed, and were expected as a treatment reaction consisting of a massive discharge of bacteria and destruction of the sebaceous glands (Figs 2.14–2.16, see page 23). Typical reactive acne entails several spots that heal within 1 week, and this occurs frequently in the perioral area. Healing is fast because bacteria in reactive acne are already dead. High-degree reactive acne is caused by excessive irradiation from the light source but the extent of reactive acne is usually in proportion to the degree of acne severity. Excessive

Clinical assessments		
Assessment	Face (No.)	Body (No.)
Worsened	0	0
Unchanged	7	4
Improved	26	16
Markedly improved	50	31

Table 2.3 Clinical assessments

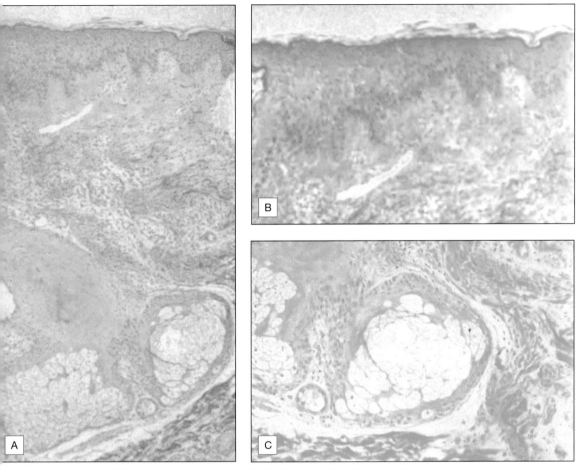

Fig. 2.4 Two days after PDT treatment to the normal skin in Figure 2.3, the damage to the sebaceous gland is seen (**C**) but the epidermis is intact (**A**, **B**)

eactive acne should be avoided because it can give ise to disfiguring acne scars. Almost all facial acne patients treated with PDT noticed reactive sebum or several days afterwards, following which they became aware of a rapid decrease in sebum. Generally, the degree of reactive sebum depends on the degree of seborrhea. Erythema, swelling, reactive acne, and reactive sebum appear most profusely after the first PDT session. On repeat PDT treatment, these reactions decrease.

The author reports a series of PDT-ALA treatments on over 5000 acne patients from 1998 to 2004. Since 1999, orally administered ALA-PDT has been the preferred route in this group, with the oral dosage used being 10 mg/kg BW. No patient has suffered from liver dysfunction (Figs 2.17–2.20, see pages 24 and 25). Five patients have developed herpes simplex on the lip within 2 d after a PDT session, but all of these patients had a past history of herpes

simplex. Among these five, two received topical ALA and three, orally administered ALA. Very frequently, hyperpigmentation and epidermal exfoliation were observed in Asian patients treated with topically applied ALA-PDT. Pigmentation change persisted over 1 week to 2 months; epidermal exfoliation lasted from the fourth to the tenth day. To avoid pigmentation and epidermal exfoliation, orally administered ALA-PDT may be preferable when treating patients with skin phototypes IV and V.

Pigmentation after topically applied ALA-PDT is caused by melanogenesis, which is a photodynamic reaction to the accumulation of PpIX in the epidermis. Pigmentation after orally administered ALA-PDT may be postinflammatory, because it is recognized in patients showing high levels of erythema and swelling. While a decrease in sebum secretion often leads to dry skin, 1 month after a PDT session, the level of sebum secretion recovers. The author has never encountered any patients with persistent, problematic photosensitivity after PDT. Adverse effects and complications are summarized in Box 2.2.

Optimal PDT treatment can lead to the eradication of etiological bacteria to acne and the suppression of new papulopustular lesions for over 6 months. Comedonal lesions are restrained because sebum is controlled. In patients with seborrhea, persistently repeated PDT procedures improve skin

---

Adverse effects and complications

After oral administration of ALA
■ Nausea and vomiting

During irradiation
■ Discomfort, burning, and stinging

After PDT
■ Erythema, swelling, 'reactive acne', 'reactive sebum', hyperpigmentation, dry skin, epidermal exfoliation (only topical application of ALA), and herpes simplex

Box 2.2 Adverse effects and complications

---

texture and decrease the secretion of sebum and pore size.

Overview of Treatment Strategy

Treatment approach

In acne patients receiving PDT, high levels of irradiation from light sources may completely eradicate bacteria in only one treatment. However complications such as erythema, swelling, reactive acne, and pigmentation, may be prominent if the irradiation is too strong. To continue treatment with no downtime, lower level irradiation is recommended for initial treatments. At subsequent PDT treatments, a step-by-step increase of the light energy is possible. For instance, if a certain patient is expected to receive four PDT treatments in one PDT series, the light energy dosage for the second PDT session may be set at 1.2 times that in the first PDT, that of the third PDT may be 1.4 times and that of the fourth 1.6 times. In a given PDT series, the number of treatments may be based on

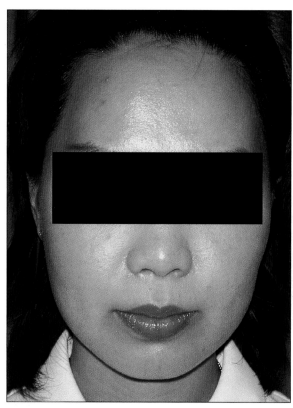

Fig. 2.5 The patient shows a very mild acne condition which was evaluated as grade I on the Burton scale. There is no treatment history

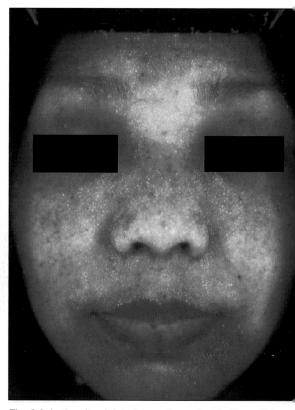

Fig. 2.6 In the ultraviolet picture, the patient in Figure 2.5 reveals an abundant fluorescence as a dot shape, which is due to endogenous coproporphyrin by *P. acnes*

he seriousness of the acne and the types of
etiological bacteria. To slightly reduce acne, two
treatments may be appropriate. However, it is
sometimes necessary to deliver treatments three
times or more. As sensitivity to PDT-ALA treatment is different for *P. acnes* compared with other
bacteria, ultraviolet examination before starting a
PDT series is important. For acne of grade IV or
more on the Burton scale, four treatment sessions
are routinely planned. In the final PDT treatment, if
reactive acne is still apparent, an additional PDT
procedure may be desired. A promising treatment
result can be expected when no more reactive acne
appears.

The interval between each PDT treatment is
usually from 10 days to 4 weeks. If a very long
interval is used, the efficiency decreases because the
bacteria propagate. If a treatment schedule is
consistent and if the skin is in reasonable condition,
an interval of 10 days is best.

For complete recovery from recurrent recalcitrant acne, treatment with only PDT-ALA may
not be sufficient, although it will show an
improvement for a time. In patients with chronic
acne, red acne scars remain for a long time even if
papulopustular lesions disappear. Moreover, a hair
follicle with redness can easily produce a papulopustular lesion again (Fig. 2.21, see page 26). If one
PDT series can stop new lesions for 6 months, the
remaining red scars should return to normal color
within this period. If the red acne scars remain
after 6 months following one PDT series, those
treated hair follicles have a likelihood of inducing
acne recurrence. To remove redness, iontophoresis
with vitamin C and intense pulsed light (IPL) treatment are effective (Figs 2.22–2.25, see page 26).
Acne scars without redness may be associated
with dimpling but do not produce recurrent acne
lesions.

PDT treatments spaced 1 month apart can reduce
sebaceous glands. However, more than 10 treatments may be necessary.

A diagram depicting the treatment approach is
shown in Figure 2.26, see page 27.

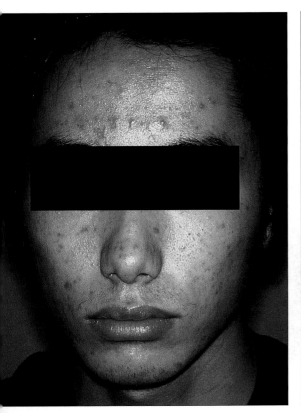

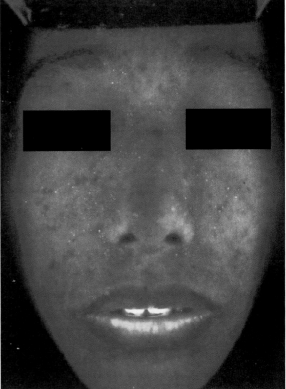

Fig. 2.7 A patient with acne of Grade IV on the Burton scale,
revealing many papulopustular lesions. The patient had
continuously undergone several typed doses of antibiotics
for 1 year

Fig. 2.8 In the ultraviolet picture, the patient in Figure 2.7
slightly reveals dot-shaped fluorescence caused by
P. acnes-based endogenous porphyrin

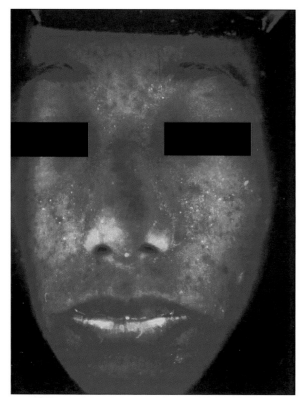

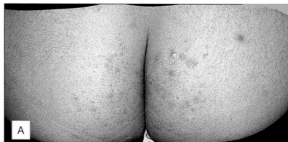

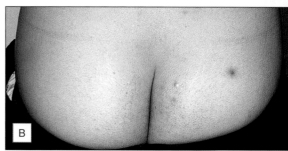

Fig. 2.10 (A) Folliculitis on the buttock. **(B)** Two weeks after two PDT sessions with a 2-week interval, the lesion shows an excellent result

Fig. 2.9 Four hours after oral administration of ALA of 10 mg/kg BW, the ultraviolet picture of the patient in Figure 2.7 demonstrates the enhancement of dot-shaped fluorescence by the accumulation of external ALA dosage-based PpIX

Patient interviews

It is important to confirm a past history of treatment:

- Have antibiotics been used?
- What was the dosage and how long was the treatment course?
- Is there a past history of herpes simplex?
- How long has the patient been suffering from acne?

A check of the skin phototype is also needed:

- Is there a history of photosensitivity?
- Is there a history of drug-induced photodermatitis?
- Is the skin seborrheic, normal, or dry?

Treatment Techniques

Patients

Acne, rosacea, seborrhea, folliculitis, and infection of the pilosebaceous units are indications for ALA-PDT treatment. Previously, application of tretinoin cream is useful to recover skin condition after PDT treatment. Medicines that could give rise to drug-induced photodermatitis should be washed out for several weeks prior to initiation of PDT. In patients with a past history of herpes simplex, a prophylactic antiviral drug should also be administered.

Equipment

The fluorescence excitation spectrum of PpIX has its peaks at: 410 nm (the Soret band), 510 nm, 545 nm, 580 nm, and 630 nm. Down to 2 mm from the surface in skin, 410 nm light provides the largest degree of photoactivation, whereas at depths exceeding 2 mm, 630 nm light is more effective. In flat normal skin, the depth of the sebaceous gland may be less than 2 mm. However, when treating highly an elevated acne papule or cystic acne, depths exceeding 2 mm are common and treatment should be using the 630 nm wavelength. Moreover, in the author's experience, compared with red light, blue light may produce stronger inflammation, erythema, swelling, and reactive acne after a PDT session.

The light source for PDT can be supplied by several types of lasers and light sources. The author

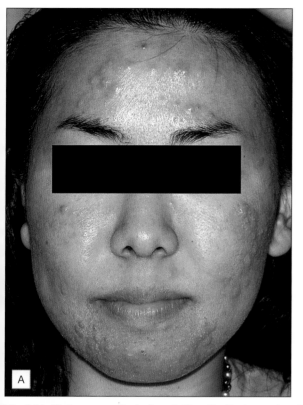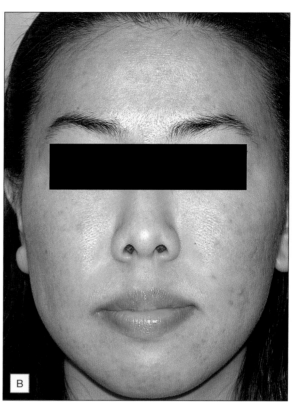

Fig. 2.11 (A) An acne patient of grade V on the Burton scale, with many papulopustular lesions and several large cystic lesions. **(B)** Three months after one PDT series (four PDT sessions), the patient demonstrates an apparent improvement

has used a 630 nm pulsed excimer dye laser (PDT-EDL 1, HAMAMATSU, Hamamatsushi, Japan) for acne treatment. However, lasers with larger spot sizes or even an incoherent light source may be more efficient at treating larger areas. Theoretically, incoherent light sources are able to produce uniform skin-surface illumination because the shape of the face is an uneven sphere, although affected areas of the chest and the back are flat. As energy density will become increased by four times if the distance between a light source and the surface of the affected area doubles, uniformity of energy density in treating large areas is very important to achieve the expected outcome. Uneven irradiation causes excessive reactive acne, erythema, swelling, hyperpigmentation, and uncertain results. It is also important that the light source be movable because it is difficult to irradiate to the region from the lower jaw to the neck if the patient is in the supine position.

At present, the author uses two light sources. One is a polychromatic visible light source with four-lamp boxes with metal halide lamps (Usio Inc.,

Tokyo, Japan; Fig. 2.27, see page 27). Although the highest peak is at 610 nm, the spectrum also efficiently covers the 545, 580 and 630 nm wavelengths absorbed by PpIX, as well as 670 nm (Fig. 2.28, see page 27). Excitation at the 670 nm peak is helpful since it too leads to the development of activated photoproducts. This device has circular spots with diameters of 5 cm and 10 cm. When the distance between the lamp and the affected surface is 13 cm, the average fluence rate and the energy-density uniformity of the light are 69.2 mW/cm^2 with a tolerance of ±11.5% using the 10 cm spot (Fig. 2.29, see page 28). The precise maneuverability of this light source permits accurate planning of treatment and makes it suitable for the treatment of facial acne.

The second light source used frequently by the author is a light-emitting diode (LED) device (Omnilux pdt, Photo therapeutics, UK), which can emit both blue and red light. LED may be the optimal light device because it is inexpensive and provides a wide irradiated area with selectively narrow wavelengths (Fig. 2.30, see page 28). The spectrum output of the red light in the authors' LED

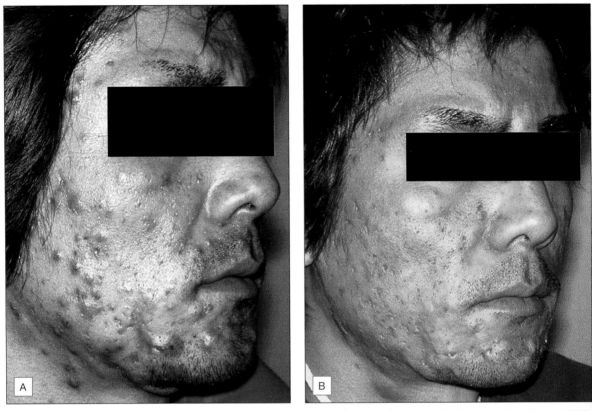

Fig. 2.12 (A) An acne patient of grade VI on the Burton scale, with many large cystic lesions. **(B)** Three months after one PDT series—four PDT sessions with 2-week intervals—the patient demonstrates an apparent improvement but deep dimples remain

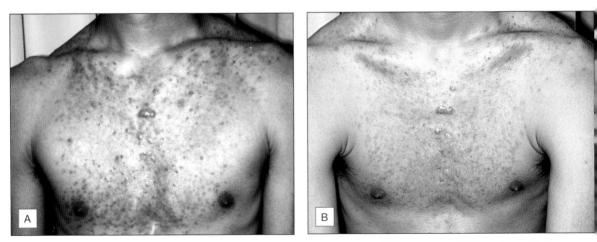

Fig. 2.13 (A) A severe acne condition on the chest. **(B)** Three months after one PDT series—two PDT sessions with 2-week intervals—the patient demonstrates an apparent improvement

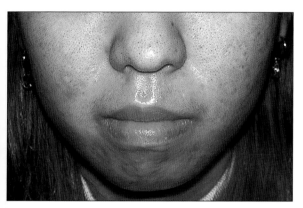

Fig. 2.14 The acne patient of grade IV on the Burton scale and the view just before the first PDT

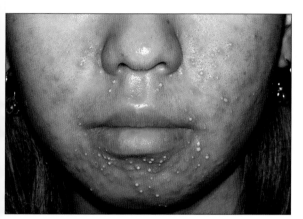

Fig. 2.15 Three days after the first PDT treatment for the patient in Figure 2.14, severe 'reactive acne' is seen. Reactive acne consists of many papules and pustules. It is caused by the irradiation being too strong. Strong irradiation is able to kill many bacteria but can produce severe reactive acne, which may lead to prolonged red acne scars. This case of reactive acne lasted for 1 week

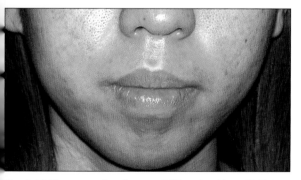

Fig. 2.16 Three months after one PDT series (three PDT treatments), the patient in Figure 2.15 demonstrates an apparent improvement. It was necessary to leave a 5-week interval between the first and second PDT because of a delay in skin recovery due to excessive reactive acne

light source (Omnilux pdt) emits along a narrow band centering on 630 nm. Because the power is high, the author usually leaves a 20 cm distance between the lamp and the target surface. Although this equipment can irradiate an extremely wide area, regrettably the energy-density uniformity can be suboptimal with an irradiation distance of 20 cm (Fig. 2.31, see page 28). Therefore, the author prefers this equipment for treating body acne because the energy dosage needed in that case is twice that for treating facial acne, and thus precision in delivered energy density is less important.

Treatment algorithm

Several weeks of pretreatment with tretinoin cream or daily iontophoresis using vitamin C derivatives is frequently used so that recovery after PDT treatment is more brisk.

Four hours after oral administration of ALA at 10 mg/kg BW, acne lesions are exposed to the light source. The ALA powder is mixed with water or orange juice for dosing. At the first PDT session, the patient should be watched in the clinic from the start of oral administration of ALA to complete irradiation because nausea is frequently observed. Nausea is almost always seen within 2 h after ALA is taken. Vomiting is rarely noted. When nausea occurs, an anti-emetic should be administered and the PDT sessions stopped for a time. However, precautionary treatment with an anti-emetic should be avoided if possible because this may impair the stability of the ALA. Starting with the second PDT session, patients may take ALA at home before coming to the clinic. Patients develop photosensitivity 2 h after oral administration. Therefore, from this time until the start of irradiation patients should stay indoors. No specific sun shielding should be prescribed, but it is preferable that clothing is dark-colored on the treatment day.

It is not necessary to use anesthesia during irradiation but the eyes, conjunctiva, lips, and mucosa must be thoroughly protected from irradiation. The total energy dose in the first PDT session with polychromatic visible light for facial acne is routinely approximately 25 J/cm². Dosages for the second, third, and fourth PDT sessions are 30, 35, and 40 J/cm², respectively. However, for serious facial acne, the first PDT session may entail only 15 J/cm², as in this condition excessive erythema, swelling, and reactive acne are often seen and can

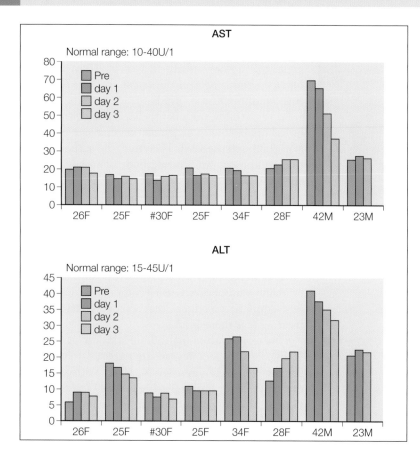

Fig. 2.17 Change over time of aspartic acid amino transferase (=GoT) and ALT at an ALA dosage of 10 mg/kg BW for two males and six females. One male patient shows a high score of AST; this patient had a history of drinking a large amount of alcohol on the night before the test. However, the AST score gets closer to the normal range day by day. # indicates a female patient who complained of nausea 2 h after oral administration of ALA

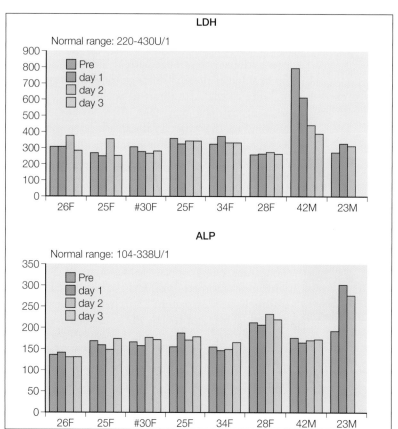

Fig. 2.18 Change over time of LDH and ALP at an ALA dosage of 10 mg/kg BW for two males and six females. One male patient shows high score of LDH; this patient had a history of drinking a large amount of alcohol on the night before the test. However, the LDH score gets closer to the normal range day by day. # as in Figure 2.17

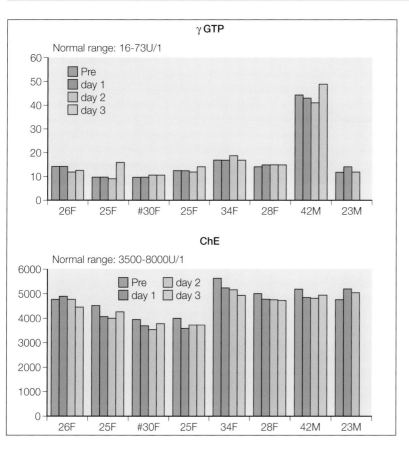

Fig. 2.19 Change over time for gamma GTP and cholinesterase at an ALA dosage of 10 /kg BW for two males and six females. All scores are within normal range. # as in Figure 2.17

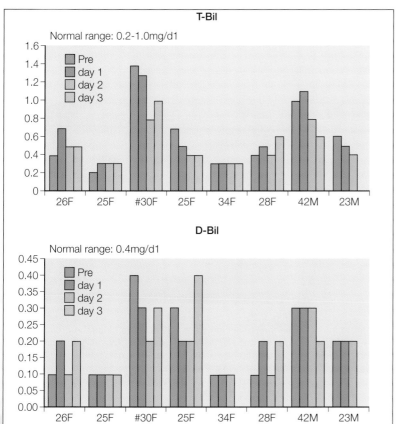

Fig. 2.20 Change over time for total and direct bilirubin at an ALA dosage of 10 mg/kg BW for two males and six females. The female patient marked #, who complained of nausea 2 h after oral administration of ALA, shows a high score of total bilirubin. However, this abnormality is already observed on the day before ALA dosage. The change after ALA dosage becomes closer to the normal range. One male patient shows a slight high score of total bilirubin. This change after ALA dosage also becomes closer to the normal range

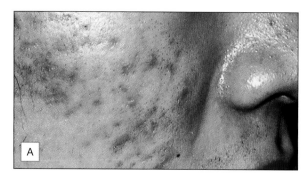
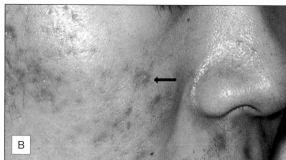

Fig. 2.21 (**A**) A red acne scar 1 week after one PDT series. There is no elective lesion. (**B**) One month later, one acne papule (arrow) is seen. This hair follicle showed a red acne scar in (**A**). The same hair follicle had a tendency to repeat papulopustular lesions

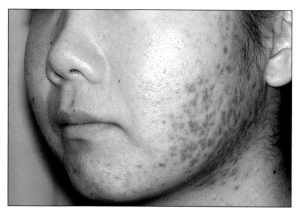

Fig. 2.22 An acne patient of grade V on the Burton scale

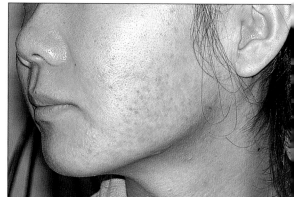

Fig. 2.24 Three months after the PDT series in the patient in Figure 2.22, discoloration of the red acne scar developed

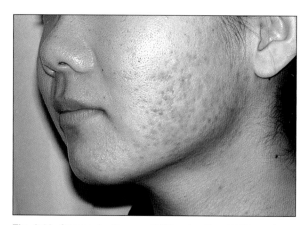

Fig. 2.23 One week after one PDT series (four PDT sessions with 2-week intervals), the affected area in the patient in Figure 2.22 shows no papulopustular lesions. The red acne scar with dimple is remarkable. The patient continues daily iontophoresis of 5% magnesium L-ascorbyl-2-phosphate solution

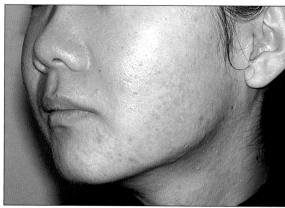

Fig. 2.25 Six months after the PDT series, the affected area in the patient in Figure 2.22 is rather close to normal skin appearance by daily iontophoresis. This skin condition is thought to be free from repeated recalcitrant acne. The dimple shown in Figure 2.22 is noted to have become flat. Compared with the old dimple, the dimple with redness is relatively easy to improve

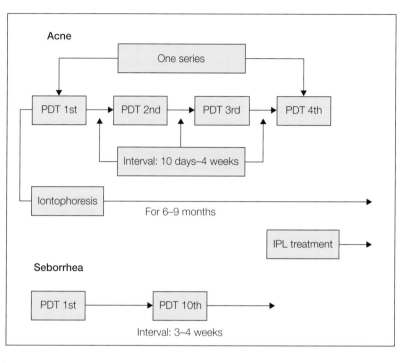

Fig. 2.26 PDT treatments for acne and seborrhea

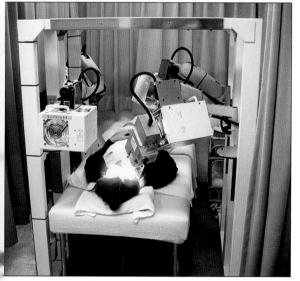

Fig. 2.27 A polychromatic visible light source with a four-lamp box by a metal halide lamp. As the movable region of each lamp box is free, it is easy to correspond to uneven regions

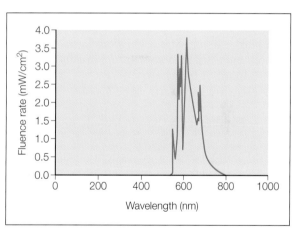

Fig. 2.28 The spectrum output of the light source in Figure 2.27 is shown. Although the highest peak is 610 nm, the wavelength efficiently covers 545, 580, 630 and 670 nm. The wavelengths of 545, 580 and 630 nm are absorbed to PpIX. As photosensitizing photoproducts with 670 nm are produced during ALA-PDT, its excitation is also advantageous

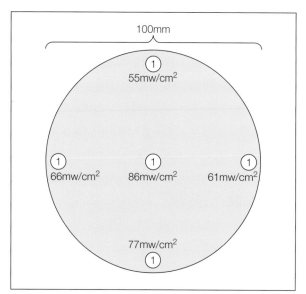

Fig. 2.29 The energy density of the light in Figure 2.27 is shown. The distance between the lamp and the affected surface is 13 cm. The average fluence rate and the energy-density uniformity of the light are 69.2 mW/cm² and an accidental error of ±11.5% on the circle area with a diameter of 10 cm, respectively

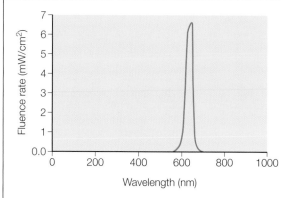

Fig. 2.30 The spectrum output of the red light in the LED light source (Omnilux) is shown. It presents a narrow band, centering on 630 nm, with high power

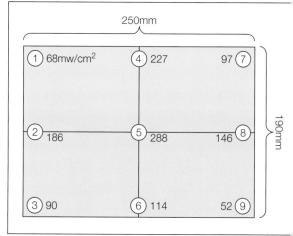

Fig. 2.31 The energy density of the light in Figure 2.30 is shown. The distance between the lamp and the affected surface is 20 cm. An accidental error of the energy-density uniformity is too large

produce severe and persistent cutaneous effects including scar formation. For body acne, the first, second, and third PDT sessions are usually at 50, 60, and 70 J/cm², respectively.

Overlap irradiation should be avoided as it causes severe reactive acne. To perform precise irradiation, the irradiated area may be divided into several parts, for example cheek, nose, and forehead.

During irradiation, most patients feel a burning sensation. If there is no such sensation, the energy density of the irradiation may be too low. If patients complain of discomfort, the energy density of the irradiation can be decreased. However, if the energy density is changed, the total energy dosage must be kept as previously scheduled. Immediately after PDT, the affected lesions show slight erythema. If there is no erythema, the energy dosage used may have been insufficient and may need to be increased.

There is almost no acne which is not affected by PDT; especially among younger patients treatment resistance is rare. If there is a fast or slower metabolizer of ALA, the starting time for irradiation will need to be changed. Usually, irradiation is started 4 hours after the oral administration of ALA. The starting time may be brought forward to 3 h after ALA dosage in younger patients. To calculate the most suitable starting time of irradiation, it is useful to take ultraviolet pictures.

After irradiation, the affected lesions are cooled for about 10 min. Cooling may be continued when the patient goes home. Sufficient cooling will decrease erythema and swelling, improving the therapeutic effects. However cooling does not decrease the occurrence of reactive acne. After PDT, make-up can be used and sun shielding on the treatment day is desirable. For 3 d after PDT, antioxidizing agents, including vitamin C and E, should be stopped. The author prefers to use daily iontophoresis of vitamin C derivatives beginning the fourth day after PDT.

Side effects, complications, and alternative approaches

Side effects and complications are summarized in Box 2.2. After the oral administration of ALA, nausea is frequently observed. When this occurs an anti-emetic and a nausea stop are prescribed for the patient. Nausea is limited to the PDT treatment day.

During irradiation, discomfort, burning, and stinging are observed. If patients do not tolerate the light irradiation, decreasing the energy density of irradiation may solve this problem.

Almost all patients develop erythema immediately after PDT treatment. Although erythema and swelling are not usually worrisome, if strong reactive acne does occur, cooling immediately after facial PDT is important and results in a decrease in erythema and swelling. Excessive reactive acne can lead to an acne scar. To avoid this problem, an energy density that is too strong and energy dosage that is too large should be avoided. The PDT operator has to pay attention to the degree of erythema, burning, and stinging during irradiation, and should change the intensity if needed.

Daily iontophoresis with vitamin C derivatives may be effective for treating excessive reactive acne and swelling, and for post-inflammatory pigmentation. Furthermore, an oral corticosteroid can be tried.

Although the irradiated light does not contain ultraviolet frequencies, immunosuppression induced by the light may cause herpes simplex. Iontophoresis with vitamin C has been reported to be effective for recovery of immunoactivity.

Iontophoresis with vitamin C

The ALA-PDT technique is fairly certain to eradicate etiological bacteria and can also prevent new papulopustular lesions developing for a time. However, in the absence of the return of acne-associated hair follicles to their normal state, papulopustular acne lesions will recur (Fig. 2.21), and patients can never be free from chronic acne.

Red acne scars may persist in their inflammatory state for a long time. The redness in acne scars has to be treated after the bacteria have been eradicated. To return the hair follicle to a normal undiseased state, the author prefers vitamin C iontophoresis (Figs 2.22–2.25, see page 26).

L-ascorbic acid (vitamin C) modulates collagen synthesis and plays an essential role in wound healing. Moreover, it also acts as an antioxidant, suppresses melanogenesis, and reduces immunosuppression. These actions may help with skin healing after the suppression of acne by PDT by diminishing redness and dimpling associated with acne scars. L-ascorbic acid is very unstable and is easily oxidized even though its molecular weight is adequate for transcutaneous penetration. Recently, some ascorbic acid derivatives have been introduced that are stable over a long period of time. The author uses magnesium L-ascorbyl-2-phosphate, which becomes attached to lipid, but the beneficial effects of this treatment appear to be limited.

Transcutaneous iontophoresis is a technique that facilitates the transport of permeants across the skin by using an electromotive force. The underlying principles of transcutaneous iontophoresis involve the placement of two oppositely charged electrodes at appropriate sites on the skin. The drug in its ionic form is placed under the electrode bearing the same charge as the drug, and the voltage source most often supplies a constant electric current that is converted to an ionic current by oxidation-reduction reactions at the electrodes. As the ions carry this current through the skin barrier, charged molecules are repelled from the active electrode into the skin and then into the systemic circulation. This has been extensively explored as a potential means for the delivery of hydrophilic agents (Fig. 2.32).

For daily iontophoresis, patients use a handy iontophoretic device (Aquapuff, Toshiba Medical Supply Co., Tokyo, Japan; Fig. 2.33). The author believes this is of value for patients with persistent acne receiving PDT treatment.

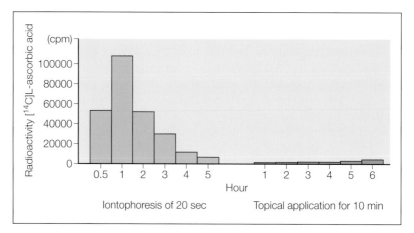

Fig. 2.32 Effect of iontophoresis on percutaneous absorption of [^{14}C] ascorbic acid in rat skin. Swabs were wetted with radioactive ascorbic acid and placed on the back skin. The iontophoretic device was immediately placed on the swabs and electric current was passed through the skin for 20 s. Swabs and electric device were removed, and then radioactive ascorbic acid remaining on the skin surface was washed exhaustively. The skins were biopsied at 0.5, 1, 2, 3, 4 and 5 h after application of ascorbic acid. The dermal layer was obtained by disperse digestion and their radioactivities were counted. For control assays, swabs were simply placed on the skin surface for 10 min instead of iontophoresis for 20 s and the skins were biopsied at 0.5, 1, 2, 3, 4 and 5 h after application of ascorbic acid. The difference between the two methods is apparent

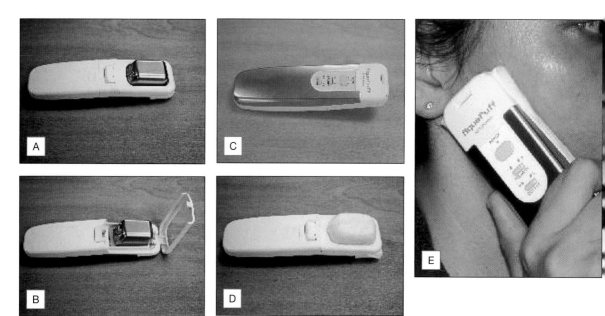

Fig. 2.33 (**A–E**) A handy iontophoretic device. The disposable cotton piece contains 5% magnesium L-ascorbyl-2-phosphate solution. Two electrodes are set up to the face and the hand

Further Reading

Cunliffe WJ, Goulden V 2000 Phototherapy and acne vulgaris. British Journal of Dermatology 142:855–856

Ebihara M, Akiyama M, Ohnishi Y et al 2003 Iontophoresis promotes percutaneous absorption of L-ascorbic acid in rat skin. Journal of Dermatological Science 32:217–222

Hongcharu W, Taylor CR, Chang Y et al 2000 Topical ALA-photodynamic therapy for the treatment of acne vulgaris. Journal of Investigative Dermatology 15:183–192

Itoh Y, Ninomiya Y, Tajima S, Ishibashi A 2000 Photodynamic therapy for acne vulgaris with topical 5-aminolevulinic acid. Archives of Dermatology 136:1093–1095

Itoh Y, Ninomiya Y, Tajima S, Ishibashi A 2001 Photodynamic therapy of acne vulgaris with topical delta-aminolevulinic acid and incoherent light in Japanese patients. British Journal of Dermatology 144:575–579

Nair V, Pillai O, Poduri R, Panchagnula R 1999 Transdermal iontophoresis. Part I: basic principles and considerations. Methods and Findings in Experimental and Clinical Pharmacology 21:139–151

Papageorgiou P, Katsambas A, Chu A 2000 Phototherapy with blue (415 nm) and red (660 nm) light in the treatment of acne vulgaris. British Journal of Dermatology 142:973–978

Tokuoka Y, Kosobe T, Kimura M, et al 2003 Photodynamic therapy for cancer cells using metal-halide lamps. Optical Review 10:116–119

Editorial

Acne Vulgaris Treated With ALA-PDT

Michael H. Gold

There is no question that Dr Yoshiyasu Itoh has compiled the largest and most impressive series of patients with acne vulgaris treated with ALA-PDT. With over 5000 cases treated with his protocols, Dr Itoh's experience truly makes him a world's expert in the treatment of acne vulgaris with ALA-PDT. The clinical results have provided much relief to these patients who have suffered intractable acne vulgaris and who have benefited from Dr Itoh's vast ALA-PDT experience.

In his chapter on the use of ALA-PDT in the treatment of acne vulgaris, Dr Itoh comments on the use of oral ALA-PDT using a 4-hour drug incubation and several light sources. He notes that topical ALA-PDT has been associated with the development of post-therapy hyperpigmentation, lasting from 1 week to 2 months after completion of the PDT. For this reason, he chooses to use oral ALA-PDT in his patient population.

We are very fortunate to have a wonderful array of medicines to treat acne vulgaris in the 21st century. These include a number of topical and oral antibiotics, topical benzoyl peroxide medicines, topical salicylic acid products, a variety of topical sulfa products as well as topical and systemic retinoids. Each group of medications has its own virtues and its own drawbacks in making one group an ideal choice for the patient suffering from acne vulgaris. Some of our topical medicines are irritating and may stain clothes. Many of the oral antibiotics have shown a high degree of drug resistance, up to 40% reported. A recent report has even suggested that the long-term use of systemic antibiotics in women may be associated with a higher incidence of breast cancer. The use of systemic retinoids may be teratogenic and has been associated with psychological problems in some individuals.

Exposure to ultraviolet light has been reported successful in treating acne vulgaris for many years. The exact mechanism for this response is not fully understood but it is felt, in part, to be the destruction of the *P. acnes* bacteria found in the sebaceous glands themselves. Chronic exposure to ultraviolet light results in photoaging and an increased incidence of skin cancers and thus precludes its regular use in the treatment of acne vulgaris.

The photodynamic reaction which is seen with the destruction of the *P. acnes* bacteria involves the natural production of porphyrins seen during the growth of *P. acnes* during the inflammatory phase of the acne cycle. The porphyrins produced are predominantly PpIX and coproporphyrin III. The absorption spectrum for these porphyrins is in the near ultraviolet range of light, in the blue range of light, with peak absorption seen at 415 nm. The PDT reaction works with exposure to an appropriate light source which will produce singlet oxygen within the *P. acnes* bacteria and ultimately destruction of the acne lesion, leaving alone surrounding tissues and structures.

Over the years a variety of light sources have been used to treat inflammatory acne vulgaris.

Recently, investigations have focused on the use of blue light sources, vascular lasers, and the intense pulsed light (IPL) sources. These lasers and light sources focus on PDT and the destruction of the *P. acnes* bacteria. Still other lasers focus on the destruction of the sebaceous gland and sebaceous gland activity output.

The use of topical 20% ALA has received a great deal of attention in the USA over the past several years as an enhancer to commonly performed laser and IPL procedures, including those for photorejuvenation and those for acne vulgaris. Elsewhere in this text is a thorough review of the current recommendations for short contact (30 min to 1 h), full-face photodynamic photorejuvenation procedures, which not only successfully treat all facets of photorejuvenation but also treat any associated AKs seen in those patients with photodamage/photoaging. Likewise, topical 20% ALA has been shown successful in enhancing a variety of laser and light sources in treating moderate to severe inflammatory acne vulgaris.

Goldman reported on the use of short-contact ALA-PDT and the IPL or blue light source in treating acne vulgaris and sebaceous gland hyperplasia. Treatments given were pain free and without any untoward effects. Relative clearing was seen in the patients after two to four weekly ALA-PDT treatments. Gold evaluated 10 patients with moderate to severe inflammatory acne vulgaris utilizing short-contact, full-face ALA-PDT and a high-intensity blue light source. Four weekly treatments showed a response rate of approximately 60% as compared to 43% with the blue light source alone in patients with mild inflammatory acne vulgaris. The treatments were tolerated well with no adverse effects and no patient downtime. Goldman and Boyce studied acne vulgaris with the blue light source with and without topical ALA in 22 individuals. They found a greater response rate in those patients receiving ALA and the blue light source than those who received blue light therapy alone. Again, the therapies were well tolerated, with no adverse events noted. Gold has reported significant clearing using ALA-PDT and a new IPL device in the treatment of moderate to severe acne vulgaris.

The combination of short-contact, full-face topical ALA therapy to enhance a variety of lasers and light sources for the treatment of acne vulgaris appears to provide a synergistic effect to effectively treat patients with moderate to severe inflammatory acne vulgaris. The combination therapy appears safe, works fast, and has not been shown to have any serious adverse effects. Post-therapy hyperpigmentation has not been seen in any of the studies thus far presented, either because of the short contact therapeutic approach now being recommended or because not enough patients have been treated for this effect to have occurred in any significant number. This is something we will have to be aware of as the USA's experience grows with topical ALA-PDT for the treatment of acne vulgaris. Topical ALA-PDT for the treatment of acne vulgaris has been evaluated by Gold in all skin types and has been shown to be useful in all those thus far studied.

ALA-PDT for the treatment of acne vulgaris is a useful and successful treatment modality utilizing a variety of lasers and light sources. More clinical research will further define the optimal parameters and devices to be used and how best to combine these new therapies with the medicines currently available for acne vulgaris.

Further Reading

Gold MH 2003 Intense pulsed light therapy for photorejuvenation enhanced with 20% aminolevulinic acid photodynamic therapy. Journal of Lasers in Medicine and Surgery 15(S):47

Gold MH 2004 A multi-center investigatory study of the treatment of mild to moderate inflammatory acne vulgaris of the face with visible blue light in comparison to topical 1% clindamycin antibiotic solution. Journal of the American Academy of Dermatology 50(S):56

Goldman MP 2003 Using 5-aminolevulinic acid to treat acne and sebaceous hyperplasia. Cosmetic Dermatology 16:57–58

Goldman MP, Boyce S 2003 A single-center study of aminolevulinic acid and 417 nm photodynamic therapy in the treatment of moderate to severe acne vulgaris. Journal of Drugs in Dermatology 2:393–396

Gollnick H, Cunliffe W, Berson D et al 2003 Management of acne: a report from a Global Alliance to Improve Outcomes in Acne. Journal of the American Academy of Dermatology 49(suppl 1): S1–S37

Leyden JJ 1997 Therapy for acne vulgaris. New England Journal of Medicine 336:1156–1162

Sigurdsson V, Krulst AC, van Weelden H et al 1997 Phototherapy of acne vulgaris with visible light. Dermatology 194:256–260

Velicer CM, Heckbert SR, Lampe JW et al 2004 Antibiotic use in relation to the risk of breast cancer. Journal of the American Medical Association 291:827–835

3

ALA-PDT Treatment of Pre-skin Cancer

Joyce B. Farah, James Ralston,
Nathalie C. Zeitouni, Allan R. Oseroff

Introduction

The problem being treated

This chapter will discuss topical photodynamic therapy for actinic keratoses (AK). Therapeutic approaches for both thin and hyperkeratotic AK will be described including aminolevulinic acid application times, skin preparation techniques, and currently available light sources.

Actinic Keratoses

Actinic keratoses are common pre-malignant lesions occurring predominantly in individuals with Fitzpatrick skin types I–III (Table 3.1). High-risk individuals have a significant history of sun exposure, and may perform outdoor professional or recreational activities, or reside in sunny climates with low latitudes where UV exposure is significant. The estimated prevalence of AKs is less than 10% in the third decade, increasing to approximately 80% by the seventh decade. Although rare, young individuals in their 20s and 30s can present with clinically typical lesions, and 60% of predisposed individuals 40 years old and older have at least one AK. Patients who have received solid organ trans-plants, or who are chronically immunosuppressed are also at greater risk for developing AK.

Although traditionally considered precancerous, AK represent points on a continuum of histological and biological change towards squamous cell carcinoma (SCC). Histologically, acanthosis, parakeratosis, dyskeratoses, and cellular atypia with mitotic figures are commonly present. It is estimated that approximately one in 20 lesions will progress to invasive carcinoma. Individuals with more than 10 AK have about a 14% probability of developing a SCC within 5 years. Because of the difficulty of predicting which lesions will become invasive, the general consensus is that all AKs should be treated. Keratinocytic intraepidermal neoplasia (KIN) has been proposed by Cockerell to represent the continuous progression from AK to SCC. The grading is analogous to the cervical intraepithelial neoplasia (CIN) nomenclature used in gynecology. KIN I is the earliest lesion that is clinically detectable with KIN III (SCC in situ) being the most advanced form with atypical cells still confined to the epidermis.

Clinical Presentation

The clinical presentation of AK ranges from a slightly erythematous scaly papule to a firm hyperkeratotic plaque. Occasionally, AK may be pigmented. Occurring on chronically sun-exposed skin, the lesions are predominantly located on the scalp, face, dorsal hands, lower extremities, and dorsa of the feet. Patients may find them asymptomatic, or may complain of burning, pruritus, tenderness or bleeding. A change in lesion character such as an increase in size, thickness or erythema, or development of ulceration is an indication for biopsy (Fig. 3.1).

AKs may also present as cutaneous horns, actinic cheilitis, or lichen-planus-like keratosis. In addition

Fitzpatrick skin types	
Skin type	**History of sun exposure**
I	Never tans and always burns
II	Tans minimally and always burns
III	Tans gradually after burning initially
IV	Tans well and burns minimally
V	Tans darkly and rarely burns
VI	Tans black and never burns

Table 3.1 Fitzpatrick skin types

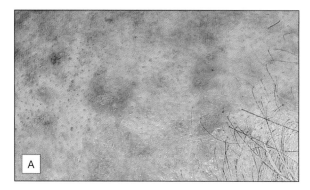

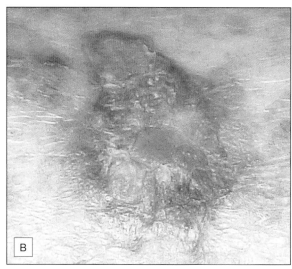

Fig. 3.1 (**A**) Thin AK on the scalp, with erythema and minimal scaling. (**B**) Hyperkeratotic and hypertrophic AK on the lower leg, with thick scaling overlying an erythematous base

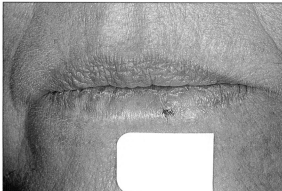

Fig. 3.2 Actinic cheilitis of the lower lip at the time of biopsy

to occurring on AKs, an estimated 16% of cutaneous horns overlie SCCs; they can also occur on a seborrheic keratosis, inverted follicular keratosis, tricholemmoma or verruca. Since it is often difficult clinically to distinguish what is underlying the cutaneous horn, a biopsy generally is required for definitive diagnoses. Actinic cheilitis most commonly involves the lower lip. Clinically, there is scaling, fissuring and/or swelling (Fig. 3.2). Painful erosions also may occur. A biopsy should be performed on any thickened area that does not heal to rule out a more invasive process. Lichen planus-like keratoses, or benign lichenoid keratoses present as erythematous to violaceous discrete lesions with a thin overlying scale. Histologically, features of lichen planus are present with focal parakeratosis.

Histopathology

Focal parakeratosis, hypogranulosis, and atypical keratinocytes are confined to the lower third of the epidermis. The epidermis can be acanthotic or atrophic. The rete ridges often form irregular downward buds (a 'budding down' appearance). Dermal changes include solar elastosis. There are thickened, serpiginous fibers that appear basophilic on hematoxylin and eosin sections, or clumps of elastotic material in which the outline of individual fibers is lost. There is typically a mild, chronic inflammatory cell infiltrate in the upper dermis. Pigmented AKs have all the features of common actinic keratoses with excess melanin in both the keratinocytes and melanocytes. Melanophages may also be present in the dermis. Actinic cheilitis features are those of an AK. There is alternating ortho- and parakeratosis in the stratum corneum. The epidermis may be acanthotic or atrophic. There may be atypical keratinocytes, disordered maturation of the epidermis and increased mitotic activity. The dermal changes include a mild to moderate chronic inflammatory cell infiltrate. Plasma cells are usually more prominent due to the involvement of the mucous membranes. Lichen planus-like keratosis has a brisk lichenoid reaction pattern with numerous Civatte bodies in the basal layer and accompanying mild vacuolar alteration. The inflammation is quite dense and is mostly lymphocytic but can have plasma cells and a number of eosinophils. The inflammation can often obscure the dermoepidermal junction. Pigment incontinence is not unusual. There is usually some hyperkeratosis and focal parakeratosis (Fig. 3.3).

Rationale for ALA-PDT Treatment

Background

The basic principles of aminolevulinic acid (ALA) photodynamic therapy (PDT) have been covered in

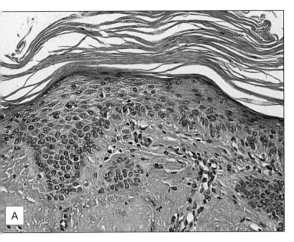

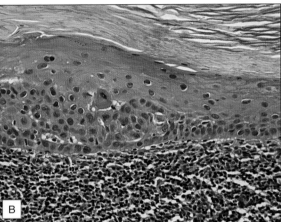

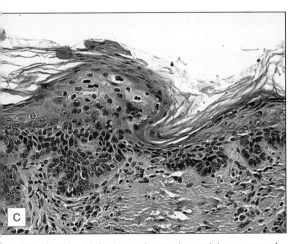

Fig. 3.3 **(A)** AK, with focal parakeratosis overlying a zone of epithelial dysplasia with a diminished granular cell zone. The dermis exhibits severe elastosis (H&E, 200×). **(B)** Pigmented AK, with focal parakeratosis associated with epithelial dysplasia, prominent pigmentation of the basal cell zone and dermal pigment incontinence (H&E, 200×). **(C)** Lichenoid AK, with focal parakeratosis, epithelial dysplasia and single cell dyskeratosis associated with a dense dermal lichenoid mononuclear cell infiltrate (H&E, 200×). (Figures provided by Dr Richard Cheney, Roswell Park Cancer Institute)

other chapters. In brief, topical ALA-PDT involves the penetration of the prodrug ALA through the stratum corneum barrier layer of the epidermis to the viable target cells, the in situ biosynthesis of the photosensitizer protoporphyrin IX (PpIX), and the subsequent photoactivation of PpIX to cause therapeutic phototoxicity by the conversion of molecular oxygen into singlet oxygen.

PDT dosimetry

The concepts of PDT dose and PDT dose rate are critical to understanding the different approaches to therapy. PDT depends on the production of singlet oxygen, and the amount of singlet oxygen produced in and around the lesion principally determines the outcome of the therapy. If there are adequate tissue levels of molecular oxygen, the PDT dose is proportional to the product of {the local concentration of PpIX} × {the delivered light dose at wavelengths that can be absorbed by the PpIX}. In the simplest approximation, the PDT dose rate, or the rate of formation of singlet oxygen, is proportional to the light dose rate (irradiance).

A particular PDT dose can be achieved with high PpIX concentrations and relatively low light doses, or vice versa, or with moderate levels of each component. Because the PpIX is eventually destroyed (photobleached) during PDT, there is an upper limit on the maximum PDT dose that can be achieved with any PpIX concentration, and a limit to the amount of useful light that can be delivered.

PpIX concentration

Since it is biosynthesized from ALA, the amount of PpIX depends on both the penetration of ALA through the stratum corneum to the viable epidermal cells, and the length of time the ALA has been applied to the skin. ALA penetration is affected by the thickness and integrity of the stratum corneum, and can be manipulated by measures taken to modify the stratum corneum and enhance drug transport.

Light dose

The size of the effective light dose depends both on the amount of delivered light, and the extent that it includes wavelengths that are absorbed by PpIX. As shown in Figure 3.4, significant PpIX absorption bands are around 410, 505, 540, 580, and 635 nm.

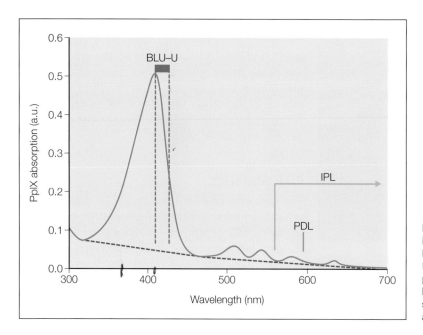

Fig. 3.4 Absorption spectrum of PpIX in a biological environment. The wavelengths produced by the BLU-U, the IPL (560 nm filter), and the 595 nm pulsed-dye laser are indicated. (The brown dashed line represents nonspecific light scattering; the PpIX absorbance is above this line)

The Soret band absorption at 410 nm is up to 15–30-fold greater than the longer wavelength 'Q bands'. Thus, for thin epidermal lesions the most effective light sources are the BLU-U (DUSA Pharmaceuticals, Wilmington MA) and the ClearLight (Lumenis Inc, Santa Clara, CA) because their output is matched to the PpIX Soret band. These sources are somewhat less effective for hyperkeratotic lesions because short-wavelength light is strongly scattered, or for pigmented lesions or skin (because of increased melanin absorption). For the same delivered light dose, longer wavelength light targeting the Q bands is less efficient because it is less well absorbed; 10 J/cm^2 at 410 nm is equivalent to 200–300 J/cm^2 at 580 or 635 nm.

The FDA-approved PDT treatment of AK uses 20% ALA in an alcohol–water solution (Levulan Kerastick, DUSA Pharmaceuticals, Wilmington, MA) applied without occlusion to nonhypertrophic AK of the face and scalp for 14–18 h. The prolonged application leads to high levels of PpIX. Illumination is with the BLU-U Blue Light Photodynamic Therapy Illuminator at 417 ± 5 nm, with a delivered dose of 10 J/cm^2, administered at 10mW/cm^2 for 16 min and 40 s. As noted earlier, this is a high light dose. Thus, with both high PpIX and light levels, approved treatment delivers a large PDT dose at a rapid rate. While the treatment conditions are efficacious according to Jeffes et al and Piacquadio et al, they can also cause discomfort. Pain from ALA-PDT is proportional to the PDT dose rate and dose, and probably is due to direct photodynamic injury to the cutaneous nerves. The pain is also proportional to the surface area treated. With the FDA-approved conditions, PDT-induced discomfort generally limits treatment to individual AK, rather than to the whole face or scalp.

Recently it has become evident that AK can respond to relatively low PDT doses, in contrast to the treatment of skin cancers, where high PDT doses appear necessary for a durable complete response (Oseroff et al). Thus, there have been multiple approaches to decreasing the PDT dose. As yet, there is no clear consensus either on the best approach, or on the minimum dose. If the dose is too low, multiple treatments become necessary, but in some circumstances this also can be desirable, by reducing the morbidity of each treatment.

The PDT dose can be reduced by decreasing either the PpIX level or the absorbed light, or both. Levels of biosynthesized PpIX increase with ALA application times. In addition, skin preparation techniques that affect the stratum corneum permeability to ALA and the possible use of occlusion, are particularly important with short applications. The light dose is dominated by the choice of light source. The three major sources in the USA are the BLU-U (or Clearlight), the pulsed-dye laser (PDL), and the intense pulsed light (IPL). A red light (570–670 nm or 590–690 nm) is used to a lesser

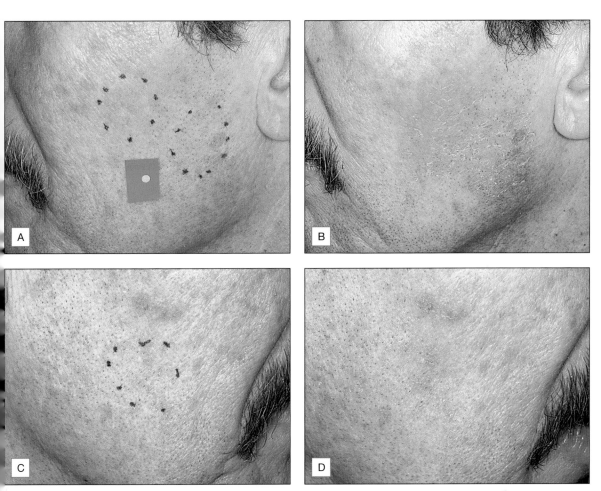

Fig. 3.5 57-year-old man with Levulan applied to individual AK for 1 h or 24 h followed by Vbeam treatment, with the clinical reactions 4 d later. (**A**) Left side before PDT. (**B**) Reaction to 24 h ALA application. (**C**) Right side before PDT. (**D**) Minimal reaction to 1 h ALA application and light

extent in the USA and more commonly in Europe for AK. As evident from Figure 3.4, blue lights are very efficiently absorbed by PpIX and would be expected to be effective even with small amounts of photosensitizer. In contrast, at 595 nm the PDL (e.g. Candela Vbeam laser) does not lie on a PpIX absorption band and is relatively weakly absorbed. With the Vbeam, higher levels of PpIX may be desirable. When operated with a 560 nm short wavelength cut-off filter, the IPL emits light from 560–1200 nm, with about 70% of the energy below 700 nm. Only about 10–15% of the IPL output is utilized by the 580 and 635 nm PpIX absorption bands, and, as with the PDL, higher levels of PpIX may be necessary to get an effective PDT dose. A 570–670 nm red lamp (e.g. Photocure CureLamp or Waldmann 1200) may have about 40–50% of its

output utilized for PpIX absorption. In summary, because the amount of singlet oxygen produced depends both on the PpIX concentration and the amount of light absorbed by the drug, it is essential to consider skin preparation, ALA application time, light source and delivered light dose in evaluating and understanding different, often equivalent approaches to treatment. Figure 3.5 shows an example of the effect of ALA application time in a patient spot-treated for thin AK on the face. The patient had 1-hour Levulan application to one side and 24-hour application to the contralateral side, followed by Vbeam therapy at a sub-purpuric light dose of 7.5 J/cm^2 in single 6 ms pulse, using a 10 mm spot size. As can be seen at the 4-day follow up, there is a more vigorous reaction with erythema and desquamation at the 24-hour application site.

Patient Selection

Patients of either sex with multiple, thin AK on the face and scalp respond best to ALA-PDT. Individuals who have failed or are intolerant of other therapies should be considered for treatment. Immunosuppressed patients or individuals with genodermatoses such as xeroderma pigmentosum also may benefit, since large areas can be treated repeatedly with minimal morbidity such as scarring or infection. While durable clinical clearance rates are lower than in matched immunocompetent controls in immunosuppressed patients, ALA-PDT can be an effective maintenance therapy. A recent study by Dragieva of transplant recipients found good tolerability of ALA-PDT with minimal morbidity and excellent cosmesis. There were no reported cases of infection. Pain was of concern but resolved shortly after cessation of therapy. As expected, hyperkeratotic lesions did not respond as well. Overall pooled complete clearance rates (CCRs) for all anatomic areas treated were 86% at 1 month, 68% at 3 months, 55% at 4 months, and 48% at 1 year.

Patients with type IV–V skin should be treated with caution due to the increased risk of developing post-inflammatory hyperpigmentation. Patients who recently received other topical therapies should not be treated with ALA-PDT until the erythema and inflammation have subsided. Exclusion criteria include porphyria or known hypersensitivity to porphyrins, known photosensitivity diseases, concurrent use of photosensitizer drugs, or women who are pregnant or lactating. Patients who are suntanned must have treatment with ALA-PDT delayed until the tan fades to avoid blistering, hypopigmentation, and decreased efficacy (Table 3.2).

Expected benefits

The efficacy of treatment is assessed by the number and/or percent of AK cleared, both as a fraction of the total AK in all patients in a study, or as the percent of patients that achieve some benchmark such as 75% or 100% clearance. The response of an AK to ALA-PDT will depend on thickness, size and location of the lesion. Complete response rates on the face and scalp are higher than on the extremities, and the larger and more keratotic the lesion, the less likely it will completely clear with a single treatment. Outcomes also depend on the treatment parameters; more aggressive treatments usually will give better outcomes, while also increasing side effects. In general, as discussed in more detail later, the response rates for individual lesions and for all AKs on a patient may range from 50–100%. Many patients require at least two treatments for complete resolution. Symptoms and erythema generally resolve with a single treatment, while hyperkeratosis and scaling are the most persistent. The durability of the response over time is also a measure of efficacy. The more effective the treatment, the longer the area will stay clear. Two months is probably the minimum follow-up interval to assess durability. A summary of results for ALA-PDT using different treatment conditions is given in Table 3.3.

In 1997, DUSA completed two multicenter Levulan PDT Phase III studies on over 1500 AK lesions in 243 patients. The patients were treated with either 20% Levulan topical solution, or a placebo vehicle, plus blue light. Patients whose lesions did not clear completely were retreated after 8 weeks. In one of the studies (117 patients), 86% of the AK lesions responded completely after a

Patient selection and exclusion criteria	
Selection criteria	**Exclusion criteria**
Multiple AKs from chronic sun exposure, immunosuppression or organ transplant, or xeroderma pigmentosum	Patients with photosensitivity diseases, porphyria or known hypersensitivity to porphyrins, or current use of photosensitizing drugs
Thin lesions, which will respond better than those with hyperkeratotic lesions	Pregnant or lactating patients
Patients with large or multiple AK who have failed other therapies or are intolerant to topical chemotherapeutic agents	Patients treated with other topical therapies until the erythema and inflammation have subsided
	Patients with suntans until the tan fades, or with type IV–V skin

Table 3.2 Patient selection and exclusion criteria

single treatment with Levulan PDT, with 94% clearing after two treatments compared with 32% clearance after two treatments with placebo and light. In the other study (126 patients), 81% of the AK lesions responded completely after a single treatment with Levulan PDT, with 90% clearing after two treatments, compared with 20% clearance after two placebo and light treatments. When the results of the two studies were combined, over 90% of the lesions had cleared after one or two Levulan

PDT treatments, compared to 25% in control groups. All of these results were highly significant statistically ($P < 0.001$).

Jeffes et al published the first investigator-blinded, randomized, vehicle-controlled study investigating the treatment of multiple nonhyperkeratotic AK of the face and scalp with topical 20% ALA and a blue light source, after a 14–18-hour application time. The investigators used 2, 5 and 10 J/cm^2. They found the higher light doses to be

	Results using different application times and light sources for AK treatment					
Application Time (h)	Light Source	Investigators	Sites	Average AK complete response rate (%)	Number of Tx	Length of follow up (months)
14–18	BLU-U	Jeffes et al, 2001	Face or scalp	85	1–2	4
14–18	BLU-U	Piacquadio et al, 2004	Face or scalp	83/91 lesions; 60/73 patients	1–2	3
14–18	PDL 1–4 pulses	Alexiades-Armenakas et al, 2003	Face or scalp	92	1	4
14–18	PDL 1–2 pulses	Oseroff et al (unpublished)	Face or scalp	85	1	4
3–4	PDL 1–4 pulses	Alexiades-Armenakas et al, 2003	Face or scalp	84	1	4
3	570–670 nm lamp	Szeimis et al, 2002 (Metvix)	Face, scalp, other	69	1	3
3	570–670 nm lamp	Pariser et al, 2003 (Metvix)	Face or scalp	89	2	3
3	570–670 nm lamp	Freeman et al, 2004 (Metvix)	Face or scalp	91	1	3
1–3	BLU-U	Touma et al, 2004	Face or scalp	93 (1 h) 84 (2 h) 90 (3 h)	1	1
1	BLU-U	Smith et al, 2003	Face or scalp	80	2	1
1	PDL 2 pulses	Smith et al, 2003	Face or scalp	50	2	1
1	IPL	Avram et al, 2004	Face	68	1	3
1	Chemolum patch 430–515 nm 0.17 J/cm^2	Zelickson (unpublished)	Face	36–100 (range of patient responses)	2	3

Table 3.3 Results using different application times and light sources for AK treatment

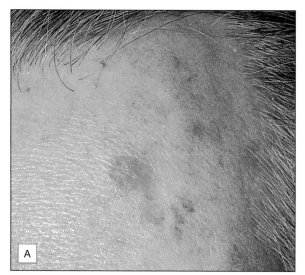 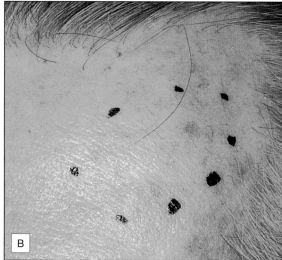

Fig. 3.6 (**A**) 63-year-old man with an AK on the forehead. (**B**) Appearance 1 year after Levulan BLU-U PDT

more effective, with complete clearing of 85% of lesions at the end of 16 weeks. Piacquadio et al, in a multicenter investigator-blinded study using ALA vs. vehicle and BLU-U, found 77% of patients had a 75% response rate at 8 weeks (75% of AKs cleared). Patients who did not achieve 75% clearance at 8 weeks were retreated; the 75% clearance rate was found in 89% of patients at 12 weeks. At 8 and 12 weeks, 66% and 73% of the patients, respectively, achieved 100% AK clearances. An example of overnight ALA and BLU-U treatment is shown in Figures 3.6A and B. The treatment was well tolerated with excellent cosmetic results; the complete clinical response was durable at 1-year follow up.

Much of the current use of Levulan involves lower PDT doses than in the original studies, from pulsed light sources and/or shorter application times. The lower doses have made it feasible to treat entire anatomic areas such as the face, rather than individual AK. In a large, single-center study, Alexiades-Armenakas et al used the 595 nm PDL (1–4 pulses) and both 14–18 and 3 h ALA application times. The 3 h ALA application was occluded to increase uptake, and hyperkeratotic lesions were covered with surgical lubricant jelly prior to laser treatment to reduce light scattering. AK responses were stratified according to anatomic site. At 4 months, the average clearance rates were 93% head, 71% extremities, and 65% trunk. The 14–18 h applications were somewhat more effective than the

3 h applications, with about an 8% greater response rate on the face and a 16% greater rate on the extremities, consistent with the difference in PDT dose, though the number of patients treated with the shorter application time was small. The lesions that did not respond tended to be >2 mm and hyperkeratotic. All nonresponding lesions were biopsied, and 69% were SCCs.

At the current authors' institution, 18–24 Levulan application has been used followed by multiple spot or confluent treatment at 595 nm with a pulsed-dye laser (Candela Vbeam) in 14 patients with 46 different anatomic areas affected. Hypertrophic lesions are pretreated with gentle abrasion with 3M Red Dot EKG tape. The entire anatomic area is single pulsed, and hypertrophic lesions are double pulsed. For a single treatment with 18–24-hour application, on a response per patient basis, the current authors found about an 80% overall CCR rate (range 60–100%) for the face and the scalp, about a 65% overall CCR rate (range 60–70%) for the upper extremities, and about a 55% CCR rate (range 30–70%) on the lower extremities. On a response per lesion basis, the face and scalp had an 85% CCR rate (Table 3.3). There was no significant pain, and mild erythema and edema typically resolved within a week. The current authors also use 4-hour ALA applications, but find this regime less effective except on the lip or mucosal surfaces. Figure 3.7 shows a 45-year-old woman with Type I skin at initial evaluation (A). Marked erythema and

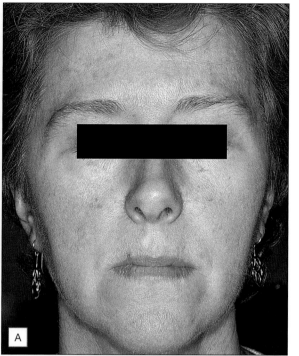

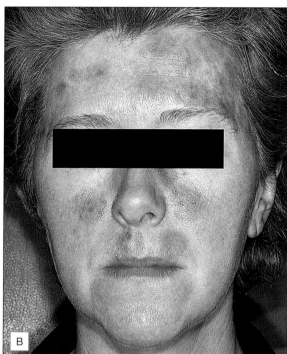

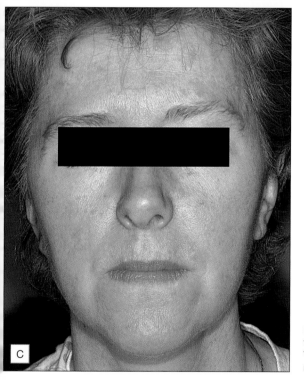

Fig. 3.7 (**A**) 45-year-old woman with Type I skin before treatment. (**B**) Immediately after 24 h Levulan application and Vbeam treatment. (**C**) At 1 week follow up, with erythema resolved

some edema is apparent immediately after spot treatment with 24-hour Levulan and Vbeam PDL irradiation, despite premedication with diphenhydramine (B). The treatment reaction largely has resolved 1 week later (C).

Several other studies have investigated short application times. Using the BLU-U in a small number of patients, Touma et al found no statistically significant difference between 1-, 2-, and 3-hour ALA applications in clearing of AK. An 'acid mantle' cream was applied to the skin for 45 min before light treatment, which may have increased the ALA uptake. Their average 90% lesion CCR rate with 1- and 5-month follow ups was comparable to the trials assessing 14–18-hour applications. They also found a modest but significant improvement in the Griffith score as well as in fine wrinkling (Table 3.3). Smith et al investigated the efficacy of 1-hour application PDT using both the BLU-U and a 595 nm PDL, compared to treatment with 5-FU. Patients were treated twice at 30-day intervals. Hyperkeratotic lesions were excluded. The patients were assessed at 1 month post-treatment and the cumulative clearance rate or individual AK lesion response rate was found to be 79%, 80%, and 60% for 5-FU, BLU-U, and PDL-PDT, respectively. The 5-FU and BLU-U groups experienced enhanced improvements in tactile roughness whereas the 5-FU and PDL group had better response in terms of pigmentation. Avram et al studied the efficacy of the IPL in treating both AK and photodamage. A total of 17 patients with greater than 3 AK and signs of photodamage on the face had Levulan applied for 1 h followed by IPL therapy using a 560 nm filter and double pulse of 3.0 ms and 6.0 ms with a 10 ms delay. Of all AK, 68% cleared after one treatment and significant improvements were seen in photodamage scores. In a very interesting preliminary study of very low-dose PDT, Zelickson used 1-hour ALA application with low-intensity chemoluminescent patches delivering a total light dose of only 0.17 J/cm², 430–515 nm. He found individual patient responses ranging from 36–100% (Table 3.3 on page 39).

The methyl ester of ALA, Metvix, methyl 5-aminolevulinate (PhotoCure ASA, Oslo, Norway) is a topical photosensitizer approved in Europe for treatment of AKs. The more hydrophobic methyl ester may have increased skin penetration, though it requires conversion to ALA by tissue esterases for activity. Pariser et al used Metvix to treat AK on

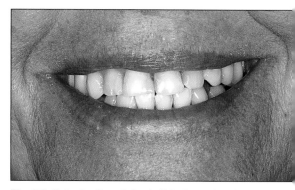

Fig. 3.8 Patient with actinic cheilitis 6 months after one treatment with Levulan and Vbeam laser. The pre-treatment image is Figure 3.2

the face and scalp after a 3-hour application with a red light source (570–670 nm). Individual lesions were pretreated with gentle curettage, and Metvix applied under occlusion. A response rate of 89% was found after two treatments, at a 3-month follow up; the CCR rate for placebo PDT was 38%. Freeman et al found similar results in a study comparing Metvix-PDT with cryotherapy. In contrast, Szeimis et al had a 69% response for lesions treated on the face, scalp and other locations after one treatment at 3 months' follow up, using Metvix with a 3-hour application without pre-treatment and a 570–670 nm light. The disparity in clearance rates between the studies may be due to the number of treatments performed or the differences in pretreatment.

Although the major clinical trials have been on AKs, there have been case reports documenting efficacy in the treatment of actinic cheilitis. The high permeability of the lip to Levulan permits short application times. Our group treated a patient with short application time ALA followed by PDL illumination. Figure 3.2 shows the initial lesion and Figure 3.8 shows the complete clinical resolution of the lesion 6 months after a single treatment with excellent cosmesis.

Comfort and convenience

In contrast to topical chemotherapeutic agents, ALA-PDT does not require prolonged application of topical agents that can cause significant morbidity. The discomfort is limited to mild burning or pruritus with drug application, and pain during light therapy that resolves within 24 h. Erythema and

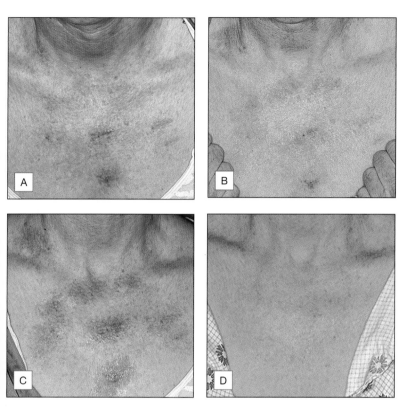

Fig. 3.9 AKs on the chest. (**A**) Before treatment. (**B**) After 24-hour Levulan application (before light). (**C**) Immediately after treatment. (**D**) At 8-month follow up

desquamation generally resolves within 7–10 d, but may extend to 4 weeks. A typical response to treatment is illustrated in Figure 3.9. The patient is a 50-year-old woman with multiple AKs on the anterior chest. Figure 3.9A shows the nonhyperkeratotic lesions at the initial visit; and Figure 3.9B shows the same area after 24-hour Levulan application, prior to laser therapy; some erythema is evident. Figure 3.9C shows the reaction immediately after PDL-PDT, and Figure 3.9D is the response 8 months after two treatments.

Cost and cost/benefit ratio

The average wholesale cost of a Levulan Kerastick is approximately $91, with a J code reimbursement of $123. One Kerastick is sufficient to cover a scalp, a face, or upper or lower extremities with two passes each. Treatments often are charged per anatomic area with the cost of the Kerastick built in. Average patient charges for a face and scalp vary with geographical location, but may range from $400–700 or more per treatment. PDT requires a light source. The BLU-U is relatively inexpensive, and the PDL and IPL have multiple uses in addition

to PDT. The overall cost of a Levulan-PDT treatment is similar to that of 5-FU or imiquimod. The typical cost for a 25 g tube of 5-FU in the form of Efudex is about $133, and an average treatment may require two tubes ($266) applied over 2–4 weeks in addition to two to four office visits. Imiquimod costs approximately $140 for a box of 12 single-use packets. A typical treatment requires three boxes of packets applied over a 12–16-week period ($420), in addition to two to four office visits. In the pivotal studies used for FDA approval of imiquimod, 45% of patients had 100% clearance and 59% had 75% clearance, so that multiple courses of treatment may be necessary.

While the costs of the wide area AK treatments are similar, there are definite benefits associated with ALA-PDT. With PDT, complete recovery may take from less than 1 week to 2 weeks, and patients may resume normal activities within a few hours of treatment. In contrast, treatment time with topical chemotherapy or immunotherapy is prolonged, and healing may take 2–4 weeks after cessation of therapy. In addition, ALA-PDT allows more physician control of the treatment and enhanced patient compliance.

Safety profile

No noncutaneous adverse events have been reported in association with ALA-PDT for the treatment of AKs. The most common recorded reactions are stinging or burning and pain during light treatment. The pain is mild to moderate and occasionally severe, depending on the patient, area treated and PDT dose. Pain generally is minimal with the PDL or IPL, or with the BLU-U and short ALA applications. The most common reaction after treatment is erythema, mild edema and desquamation that resolves in 1–2 weeks. The reaction can be significant: Figure 3.10A shows a facial AK on a 65-year-old man before 24 h Levulan application. Figure 3.10B shows a severe erythematous edematous reaction after PDL-PDT with the Vbeam laser. Crusting purpura or scarring are very rare occurrences. Particularly after prolonged application ALA-induced PpIX in the skin can cause phototoxic reactions from ambient light exposure before treatment, ranging from mild erythema (e.g. Fig 3.9.B) to severe erythema and edema. If a pretreatment phototoxic reaction occurs, it may photobleach the PpIX so that there will not be significant additional erythematous response following light treatment. This phototoxicity generally resolves within 5–10 d.

Overview of Treatment Strategy

Topical ALA-PDT is more effective for thin AK on sun-damaged skin than for hypertrophic AK. To treat hyperkeratotic lesions or enhance ALA uptake with short application times, permeability can be increased with the various techniques described later. ALA uptake and PpIX synthesis increase with longer application times. Thin lesions may respond well to short application times while hypertrophic thick lesions may be better treated with longer ALA applications. Decisions about application times also are affected by patient comorbidities and preferences, office practice considerations and available light sources. Units that deliver higher absorbed light doses, such as the BLU-U, are more effective with shorter drug application times that result in overall lower PpIX concentrations in target cells. PDL and IPL sources delivering lower absorbed light doses may require longer times. Since our patients often have hyperkeratotic AK and tend to prefer fewer, more aggressive treatments, the current authors generally use 18–24-hour drug application followed by 595 nm Vbeam therapy.

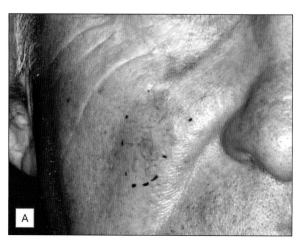

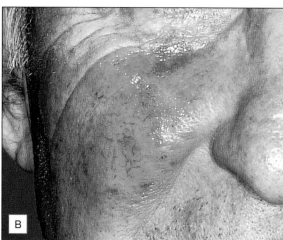

Fig. 3.10 65-year-old man. **(A)** Before treatment of AK on cheek. **(B)** Exuberant reaction immediately after therapy with PDL and 24 h Levulan application

Treatment approach and major determinants

As discussed earlier, the fundamental treatment decisions are the choices of PDT doses and dose rate, which are affected by both the light source and the ALA application time. While the PDT-induced inflammatory response probably plays a role in AK resolution and the lowest effective PDT dose has not been defined, there appears to be at least some relationship between PDT dose and outcome. There is a clear relationship between dose, dose rate and side effects, including pain. A flow chart of treatment decisions is shown in Figure 3.11.

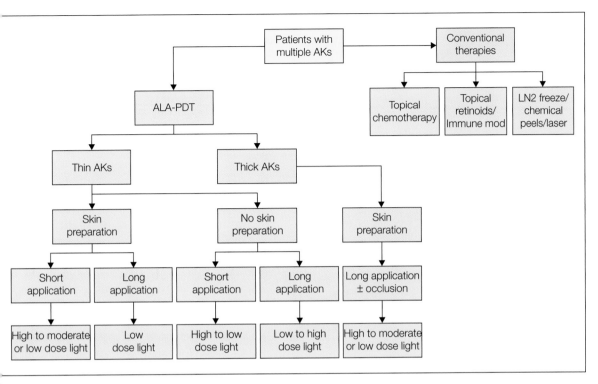

Fig. 3.11 Treatment algorithm

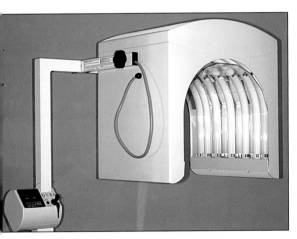

Fig. 3.12 The BLU-U. (With permission of DUSA Inc.)

reserved for spot treatments and for hyperkeratotic lesions. Shorter applications of 1–4 h allow treatment of the full face or scalp. Patients will vary in their response to PDT, and varying the application time as well as the skin preparation allows modulation of the photodynamic effect and the phototoxicity. Note that it often is not necessary to deliver the full $10\,J/cm^2$ (16.6-minute treatment). It may be adequate to periodically interrupt illumination and look at the skin, treating until there is mild erythema at the AK. Note that the shape of the BLU-U is optimized for facial and scalp lesions (Fig. 3.12). It can be used for the hands and feet, but is less practical for extremities and trunk. These areas are more easily treated with a PDL, IPL, red lamp or LED array.

BLU-U

The BLU-U is the least expensive light source. The light's output is strongly absorbed by PpIX in keratinocytes above the dermal vasculature. Thus, in most patients overnight ALA application leads to PpIX levels too high to permit full-face or scalp application, so this interval generally should be

PDL and IPL

Compared to the BLU-U, the long pulse dye laser and IPL are less efficient sources for ALA-PDT of AK, but adequate efficacy can be obtained with appropriate skin preparation and ALA application time. Again, these factors may need to be adjusted for individual patients. The time required to treat an

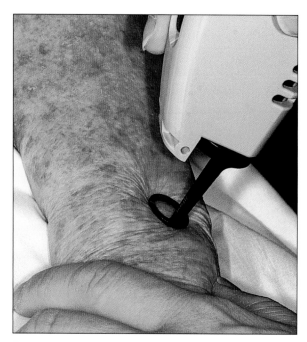

Fig. 3.13 Vbeam laser being used to treat AKs on the forearm. (With permission of Candela Corporation)

entire face can be shorter than what is used with the BLU-U with a $10\,J/cm^2$ light dose. Both the PDL and IPL can be used for a range of ALA-PDT and nonPDT indications. There currently is no available data favoring one over the other for PDT, and a choice between them would depend on other factors, including physician preference. Figure 3.13 shows the Vbeam PDL being used to treat extensively damaged skin on a forearm.

Patient interviews

The following is a sample patient questionnaire:

Extent of the problem

1. Where are your AKs located? (Face/scalp/arms/legs/body)
2. How many AKs do you have? (A few/moderate number/many)
3. Are your AKs thick or scaly? (None/some/many)

Prior therapy

4. Have you had treatment for AKs in the past? (If yes, with what?)
5. Have you had treatment in the past 2 months? (Yes/no)
6. Have you previously used 5-fluorouracil (5-FU Efudex or Carac), or Aldara? (Yes/no) If so, have you had any problems with the treatment or with healing? (Yes/no)
7. Have your lesions been treated with freezing in the past? (Yes/no) If yes, were you pleased with the result. (Yes/no)
8. Have you ever had PDT? (Yes/no)

Lifestyle preferences

9. In addition to the treatment of your AKs, are you interested in the possibility of skin rejuvenation? (Yes/no)
10. Would you like to have your whole face treated to eliminate early AKs that are too small to see and possibly reduce photoaging, or would you prefer just treatment of the visible AKs? (Visible AKs only/whole face treated)
11. Do you prefer fewer, 'stronger' treatments that may make your skin more red and take longer to heal, or a greater number of more 'gentle' treatments?
12. Can you accommodate a treatment where the medication is applied in the afternoon and you are treated the next day, or do you prefer one in which the medication is applied and you are treated after a 1–4 hour interval on the same day?
13. Do you use sunscreen? (Never/occasionally/frequently/every day)

Medical history

14. List your medications (prescription, nonprescription and any herbal supplements)
15. Do you have Lupus or an immune system disease? (Yes/no)
16. Have you had an organ transplant? (Yes/no)
17. Are you on immunosuppressive therapy? (Yes/no)
18. Do you have porphyria? (Yes/no).

Treatment Techniques

Equipment

ALA-PDT requires a standard patient examination room with appropriate light source(s) for PpIX activation. A power table is useful, but not essential. We dispense the Levulan Kerasticks. Some

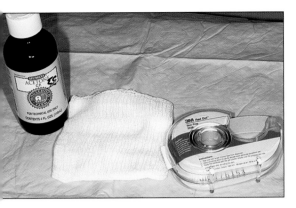

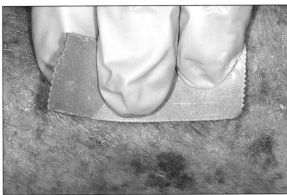

Fig. 3.14 Acetone and 3M RedDot Trace Prep 2236 tape for skin preparation. (With permission of 3M Healthcare)

Fig. 3.15 Gentle thinning of the stratum corneum with 3M EKG tape

practitioners have the patient obtain the drug by prescription from a pharmacy. One Kerastick usually is sufficient to cover a face and scalp, bilateral upper extremities, or bilateral lower extremities with two drug applications.

Patients having short application time treatments should be provided with a waiting area that has low levels of ambient light to avoid possible phototoxic reactions after ALA application.

Staffing requirements during treatment consist of a physician and a nurse or assistant. The physician generally performs the initial assessment, skin preparation and drug application. The nurse or assistant can run the BLU-U. Depending on State regulations, nurses or assistants may be able to carry out the laser treatments.

Treatment algorithm
Skin preparation prior to drug application

As previously discussed, hypertrophic lesions present a barrier to both drug and light penetration. The barrier can be decreased by removal of lipid with acetone and/or physical removal of the stratum corneum by curetting, or gently sanding the lesions with 3M Red Dot EKG tape (Fig. 3.14), or by microdermabrasion. Sanding can be done on single lesions, or alternatively, entire anatomic areas can be pretreated. Gentle pressure should be applied to avoid damage to the surrounding epidermis (Fig. 3.15). In addition, for hyperkeratotic AK, keratolytic agents such as 40% urea cream can be prescribed for use several weeks prior to drug application. According to Touma, these agents do not appear to benefit thin AK. Applying a transparent cream or gel, or mineral oil to hyperkeratotic AK prior to light

treatment will reduce light scattering and increase the effective light dose.

Drug application technique

Proper application is essential for optimal target cell PpIX accumulation. The Levulan Kerastick is composed of two crushable ampules. The bottom ampule (labeled A) contains the solution vehicle and should be crushed first. Ampule B, containing the ALA, should then be crushed starting at the top and moving down toward ampule A (Fig. 3.16). The Levulan Kerastick should be held between the thumb and forefinger with the cap pointing away from the face, and shaken gently for at least 3 min to ensure complete mixing of the contents. The cap is then removed and the drug is applied to the target lesions or entire anatomic areas by gently dabbing with the applicator tip (Fig. 3.17). Once the solution has air-dried, a repeat application should be performed. For thick or resistant lesions it may be helpful to reapply the Levulan a third time. ALA is transported into the stratum corneum only until the vehicle has dried, though additional transport will occur if the site is hydrated by occlusion. The Kerastick should not be applied to the periocular area or to mucous membranes. Once activated, the Kerastick should be discarded after 2 h.

BLU-U

The FDA-approved treatment requires two office visits on consecutive days. On day 1, the patient has the Levulan Kerastick applied to clean, dry skin. On day 2, 14–18 h later, the patient is placed under the BLU-U, with appropriate eye protection for

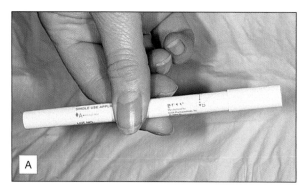

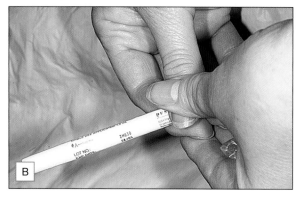

Fig. 3.16 (**A**) The Levulan Kerastick. (**B**) Crushing the Kerastick ampules. (With permission of DUSA, Inc.)

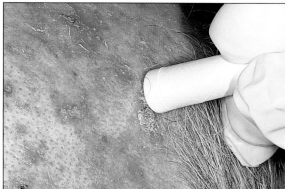

Fig. 3.17 Proper Levulan application technique with the Kerastick held perpendicular to the skin. (With permission of DUSA, Inc.)

16 min 40 s. Post-treatment, the area may show mild to severe erythema and edema. Note that as mentioned earlier, shorter treatment times (e.g. 8–12 min) may be adequate.

In contrast to the FDA-approved treatment, short duration ALA application requires only one prolonged office visit. Application times range from 1–4 h before light treatment. Longer times allow greater synthesis of PpIX, which may increase both efficacy and side effects, particularly with wide areas or high light doses. The short ALA application time BLU-U light dose used in published studies is $10 \, J/cm^2$ (16 min 40 s).

PDL

For long application times, similarly to the original approach with the BLU-U, ALA is applied overnight for 14–24 h, and the patient returns the following day for laser therapy. For short application times, ALA is applied for 1–4 h. The current authors use the Candela Vbeam laser at subpurpuric thresholds. The settings include a 10 mm spot size, 6 ms pulse duration, $7.5 \, J/cm^2$ pulse energy and cryogen spray settings of 30/10. Since patient skin type varies, it is

suggested that a test spot be performed to ensure subpurpuric light doses. Hyperkeratotic lesions can be double or triple pulsed. With this method, either entire anatomic areas or discrete lesions can be treated.

IPL

The overall approach to the IPL generally is similar to that for the PDL. For short ALA application times, it is important to maximize ALA penetration and fully utilize the available PpIX. In an approach developed by Mitchel Goldman, microdermabrasion first is performed over the area to be treated. The face is then washed with acetone on a 4×4 gauze and Levulan is applied for 60 min. The IPL treatment is performed with a 560 nm cut-off filter using a double pulse of 3.0 ms and 6.0 ms at $35 J/cm^2$ to the entire anatomic area, but avoiding the beard area in men. There is subsequent illumination with the BLU-U or the ClearLight for 10 min to photobleach the remaining PpIX (and prevent subsequent ambient light phototoxicity) and to treat areas skipped with the IPL.

Patient precautions

Patients must protect the photosensitive areas from exposure to sunlight or bright indoor lighting (examination lights, tanning booths, dental examination lamps, etc.) prior to light treatment. Broad-spectrum sunscreen offers partial protection against UVA and violet light photoactivation, but will not fully protect the patient, as it will not block visible light. The ambient light photoactivation reaction may lead to stinging, burning and erythema at the drug application sites. The patient should also be cautioned not to wash the areas after drug application and prior to light treatment. After therapy, sunscreen should be applied to the treated areas in the office prior to discharge. Patients should maintain the sun and bright light precautions for the next 24–48 h to avoid phototoxic reactions from residual PpIX. As noted earlier, after PDL or IPL treatment, some physicians photobleach residual PpIX with a brief BLU-U exposure.

Pain control measures

Patients can be given nonsteroidal anti-inflammatory drugs (NSAIDs) or acetaminophen (before and after treatment), topical anesthetics such as Emla cream (EMLA, AstraZeneca) or cooled Xylocaine gel prior to light therapy (note that EMLA cream is pH9 and ALA is unstable at pH>4.5, so EMLA should not be applied directly after Levulan). The use of dynamic cooling devices on most lasers help decrease pain and epidermal damage during treatment. For lamp illuminations, a cooling fan directed at the treatment site is very effective in decreasing discomfort. Post-therapy, patients can use ice packs and NSAIDs or acetominophen as needed. PDT will degranulate mast cells, so patients with Type I skin generally will benefit from an antihistamine such as diphenhydramine (Benadryl) prior to light therapy to decrease reactions to histamine release.

Troubleshooting

Patients have variable skin responses to ALA-PDT. Some sense of the phototoxic reaction is evident immediately after therapy, with the maximal effect peaking at 24 h. If there is inadequate treatment response and minimal phototoxicity, the PDT dose needs to be increased by either increasing the Levulan application time (if overnight application times were used), and/or giving more light. More aggressive skin preparation to increase Levulan preparation also may help. Conversely, if an exuberant reaction occurs with a laser or the patient experiences extreme discomfort with the BLU-U, the Levulan application time or the light dose may need to be decreased.

Side effects and complications

The most common side effect during treatment is a burning, stinging pain, likely due to activation of PpIX that has accumulated in cutaneous nerve endings. Nonsteroidal anti-inflammatory agents, topical anesthetics applied prior to light therapy, and cooling fans during BLU-U illumination can relieve discomfort. Additionally, cool compresses may be used immediately post-treatment to relieve pain and swelling. The pain usually subsides within 1–24 h after treatment. Because there can be damage to cutaneous nerves, some patients may notice a slight, transient decrease in sensation. In the current authors' experience, this always resolves.

The other common side effects of PDT are transient edema and a sunburn-type reaction with desquamation that usually resolves within 4 weeks. There may be damage to sebaceous glands, resulting in temporarily drier skin that can be relieved with moisturizers. With damage to the skin barrier, infection is a possible, though uncommon, complication. Routine use of either topical or oral antibiotics is not recommended. Lesions that do not respond to two treatments should be biopsied to rule out SCC.

Alternative therapies

There are a number of alternative therapies available for treating AK: physical destruction, topical chemotherapy and immune response modifiers (Table 3.4).

Cryotherapy is the most commonly used destructive method, but only is practical for a limited number of lesions. Healing usually is uneventful, but can be problematic on the lower legs; the most distressing complication is residual hypopigmentation at the treatment sites. Curettage without electrodesiccation is used for hypertrophic lesions. Topical chemotherapy is best suited for multiple diffuse lesions; the most common agents are 5-fluorouracil cream and diclofenac sodium gel. The immune response modifier imiquimod recently has been approved for AK. Its exact mechanisms of action are still unclear. The most common side effects include erythema, erosion, peeling, ulceration and eschar formation. Topical retinoids, chemical peels, and laser resurfacing have also been used for multiple AKs.

Pitfalls

The treating physician should always be aware of the following:

■ Always have a low threshold for biopsy of suspicious lesions in organ transplant recipients or immunosuppressed patients.

Available treatment methods		
Method	**Application**	**Disadvantages**
Cryosurgery	Single lesion Multiple lesions	Hypopigmentation Bullae with possible secondary infection Pain
Curettage	Single or a few lesions Hypertrophic lesions	Pain Bleeding if on blood thinners
Excision	Single lesions Not recommended	Wound healing Cosmesis
Topical chemotherapeutic agents (5-FU, Solaraze, Carac)	Diffuse disease Clinically latent disease on a background of solar elastosis	Erythema, edema, crusting, erosion Pain Length of treatment and patient compliance
Topical retinoids	Multiple lesions Clinically latent disease	Erythema and inflammation Length of treatment and patient compliance
Chemical peels/laser	Multiple lesions Diffuse disease	Prolonged healing time/pain Cost Availability
PDT	Diffuse disease	Availability Cost
Immune modifiers imiquimod	Single lesions Multiple lesions Clinically latent disease	Erythema and inflammation Cost Prolonged treatment course

Table 3.4 Available treatment methods

- Any lesion that does not heal after multiple treatments should also be biopsied.
- To avoid purpura or blistering when using the PDL or IPL, always use a test spot to confirm that you are delivering a subpurpuric light dose.
- Always consider the clinical behavior of a lesion, regardless of biopsy result. A superficial biopsy may miss a more aggressive tumor.

Conclusion

ALA-PDT for the treatment of premalignant lesions is safe and effective. It is easily accomplished in the office setting. There have been no systemic adverse events reported in association with this therapy. The added benefit of ALA-PDT is the photorejuvenation effect without adverse side effects or invasive procedures. It is cost effective when multiple lesions and broad areas can be treated. Retreatments may be required within intervals of months. Patient acceptance is high.

More controlled clinical trials are required to elucidate the optimal drug application times and light doses using the different sources available in a clinical setting.

Further Reading

Alexiades-Armenakas MR, Geronemus RG 2003 Laser-mediated photodynamic therapy of actinic keratoses. Archives of Dermatology 139:1313–1320

Avram DK, Goldman MP 2004 Effectiveness and safety of ALA-IPL in treating actinic keratoses and photodamage. Journal of Drugs in Dermatology 3:S32–S39

Cockerell CJ 2000 Histopathology of incipient intraepidermal squamous cell carcinoma ('actinic keratosis'). Journal of the American Academy of Dermatology 42:(1 Pt 2):S11–S17

Dragieva G, Hafner J, Dummer R et al 2004 Topical photodynamic therapy in the treatment of actinic keratoses and Bowen's disease in transplant recipients. Transplantation 77:115–121

Freeman M, Vinciullo C, Francis D et al 2003 A comparison of photodynamic therapy using topical methyl aminolevulinate (Metvix) with single cycle cryotherapy in patients with actinic keratosis: a prospective, randomized study. Journal of Dermatological Treatment 14:99–106

Goldman MP, Atkin DH 2003 ALA/PDT in the treatment of actinic keratosis: spot versus confluent therapy. Journal of Cosmetic and Laser Therapy 5:107–110

effes EW, McCullough JL, Weinstein GD, Kaplan R Galzer SD, Taylor JR 2001 Photodynamic therapy of actinic keratoses with topical aminolevulinic acid hydrochloride and fluorescent blue light. Journal of the American Academy of Dermatology 45:96–104

Marcus SL, McIntyre WR 2002 Photodynamic therapy systems and applications. Expert Opinion on Emerging Drugs 7:331–334

Oseroff AR, Shieh S, Frawley NP et al 2004 Treatment of diffuse basal cell carcinomas and basaloid follicular hamartomas in nevoid basal cell carcinoma syndrome by wide area ALA-PDT. Archives of Dermatology (in press)

Pariser DM, Lowe NJ, Stewart DM et al 2003 Photodynamic therapy with topical methyl aminolevulinate for actinic keratosis: Results of a prospective randomized multicenter trial. Journal of the American Academy of Dermatology 48:227–232

Perry R 2004 Current concepts in the management of actinic keratosis. Journal of Drugs in Dermatology 3:S5–S16

Piacquadio DJ, Chen DM, Farber HF et al 2004 Photodynamic therapy with aminolevulinic acid topical solution and visible blue light in the treatment of multiple actinic keratoses of the face and scalp. Archives of Dermatology 140:41–46

Smith S, Piacquadio D, Morhenn V, Atkin D, Fitzpatrick R 2003 Short incubation PDT versus 5-FU in treating actinic keratoses. Journal of Drugs in Dermatology 6:629–635

Szeimis RM, Karrer S, Radakovic-Fijan et al 2002 Photodynamic therapy using topical methyl 5-aminolevulinate compared with cryotherapy for actinic keratoses: a prospective randomized study. Journal of the American Academy of Dermatology 47:258–262

Touma D, Yaar M, Whitehead SM, Konnikow N, Glichrest BA 2004 A trial of short incubation, broad-area photodynamic therapy for facial actinic keratoses and diffuse photodamage. Archives of Dermatology 140:33–40

4

Treatment as Prevention for Skin Cancer

Catherine Maari, Robert Bissonnette

Introduction

Squamous cell carcinoma and basal cell carcinoma

Basal cell carcinoma (BCC) and cutaneous squamous cell carcinoma (SCC) are the most frequent human cancers in Caucasians. These tumors can invade adjacent structures causing local destruction, which can lead to significant cosmetic impairment. In addition SCCs and more rarely BCCs can metastasize. The incidence of both BCC and SCC is on the rise. It is estimated that almost one in three Caucasians born in the USA after 1994 will develop a BCC in their lifetime. The cost of treating these tumors has been estimated at $400 million per year for the US Medicare population alone. Sunlight exposure is the major cause of BCC and SCC. Ultraviolet B radiation (UVB) (280–320 nm) is highly mutagenic and can induce actinic keratoses (AKs) and SCC in hairless mice as well as BCC in the PTCH heterozygous mouse.

The incidence of nonmelanoma skin cancer has been increasing by 2–3% per year in the USA. It is therefore a priority to develop strategies to prevent BCCs and SCCs. This will not only reduce morbidity and mortality rates but will also decrease the financial burden on health care systems created by treating these lesions.

Current strategies for skin cancer prevention

Current skin cancer prevention strategies mostly rely on sun avoidance and sun protection with sunscreens and clothing. Frequent medical visits for patients at higher risk such as fair-skinned individuals, patients with a previous history of BCC or SCC, and organ transplant recipients are also per-formed to detect and treat early lesions. Treatment of AKs is of utmost importance in order to stop progression into invasive SCCs (see Ch. 3).

Prospective studies suggest that the regular use of sunscreens can decrease the number of new AKs and SCCs. Small open studies with patients at high risk suggest that oral retinoids can reduce the risks of developing SCC. However patients often do not tolerate oral retinoids because of their muco-cutaneous and musculoskeletal side effects. A large randomized trial by Levine with retinol or low-dose isotretinoin did not demonstrate significant chemo-preventive effects in patients with a history of at least four BCCs or SCCs.

A number of animal studies have suggested that the use of oral and/or topical antioxidants such as green tea polyphenols, and vitamins C and E can prevent the development of UV-induced actinic keratoses and SCC. A large cohort study has shown that oral supplementation with vitamins A, C and E, folate and carotenoids did not provide protection against the development of SCCs. A randomized trial involving more than 1000 patients showed that selenium supplements not only failed to prevent BCC and SCC, but actually increased the risk of developing SCC. Chemoprevention of skin cancer is a very active research field. One of the currently pursued strategies is the targeting of key molecules in the ultraviolet-light signal-transduction pathway such as the activator protein-1 and cyclooxygenase-2.

Additional preventive measures for nonmelanoma skin cancers are definitely needed in view of the limited number of options currently available. Large-surface photodynamic therapy with amino-levulinic acid has the potential to become an important skin cancer prevention modality for BCCs and SCCs.

Skin Cancer Prevention Using Photodynamic Therapy in Animal Models

Prevention of SCC

Prospective clinical studies designed to evaluate skin cancer prevention strategies are difficult to perform because of the delay between carcinogenesis induction and actual lesion appearance, ethical issues related to voluntary exposure to carcinogenic agents as well as the low incidence of new skin cancers in most populations. This situation explains why animal models, such as the hairless mouse, are frequently used to explore new skin cancer prevention methods. This immunocompetent mouse is characterized by an almost complete absence of hair, which combined with its small size and easy availability, makes it ideal for skin cancer prevention studies.

Following daily UV radiation exposure hairless mice develop skin tumors within 2–4 months. The first lesions are AKs and evolve with time into invasive SCC. The appearance of these tumors is influenced by daily UV radiation dose, UV exposure frequency, as well as the wavebands of UV radiation generated by the UV source. Most of the early studies and many current skin cancer induction studies are performed with fluorescent bulbs, the so-called FS lamps. The spectral output of these sources contains UVC, UVB and UVA radiation. Although this combination is highly carcinogenic it is not the most biologically relevant as UVC does not reach the surface of the earth. Filters should be used on these sources to filter out UVC radiation.

In skin cancer prevention experiments performed with aminolevulinic acid (ALA) photodynamic therapy (PDT), mice are usually exposed 5–7 days a week to UV radiation from fluorescent lamps. In addition they also receive weekly to monthly large-surface ALA-PDT treatments. ALA is applied on the back of mice with subsequent activation by a visible light source. Pink–red porphyrin fluorescence can be seen on hairless mouse skin after ALA application (Fig. 4.1). Light sources are placed on top of cages so that mice are free to move during both UV and light exposure. Mice are carefully examined weekly for the presence of skin tumors. Kaplan–Meier curves are used to compare the tumor-free survival of mice exposed daily to UV radiation only, to mice exposed to UV radiation and treated in addition with weekly ALA-PDT.

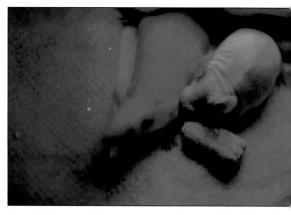

Fig. 4.1 Pink–red fluorescence can be seen with a Wood's lamp on the back of a hairless mouse (right) following ALA administration. The mouse on the left did not receive ALA

Using the hairless mouse Stender et al showed that weekly topical ALA-PDT can delay the appearance of AKs and SCC induced by chronic UV radiation exposure. However in this original report it was observed that more ALA-PDT-treated mice were withdrawn because of large tumors as compared to mice exposed only to UV radiation. The current authors' group subsequently studied systemic (intraperitoneal) weekly ALA-PDT sessions. They showed that this therapy could delay the appearance of AKs and SCCs, including the number of tumors per mouse, without inducing large tumors (Fig. 4.2).

In order to perform a study that was as close as possible to the clinical situation, the current authors exposed a group of hairless mice to UV radiation for only 8 weeks followed by weekly ALA-PDT sessions. In this experiment PDT was performed with topical ALA in the commercially available vehicle and with the Blue-U tubes. In that study chronic UV exposure took place before weekly ALA-PDT sessions were started in order to create a more clinically relevant situation where patients diagnosed with skin cancer often tend to avoid additional sun exposure. A delay in the appearance of both AKs and invasive SCC was observed (Fig. 4.3). The current authors have also repeated Stender's protocol as best as could be done, using similar UV and visible light sources but failed to see any increase in incidence of large tumors. Similar prevention studies were also performed with topical application of methylaminolevulinate (MAL) and it was again shown that mice exposed chronically to

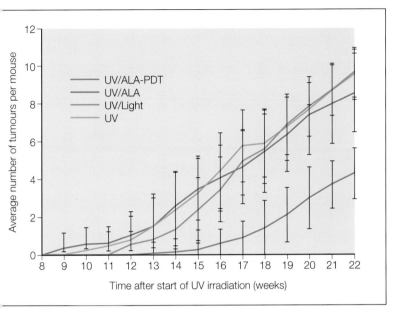

Fig. 4.2 Number of skin tumors per mouse according to time after the start of UV irradiation. Mice were exposed 5 days per week to UV radiation and treated weekly with ALA-PDT. Weekly ALA-PDT induces a delay in tumor appearance as well as a decrease in the average number of tumors per mouse. Reproduced from Sharfaei et al. Br J Dermatol 144:1207;2001 with permission from Blackwell Publishing

UV radiation and treated weekly with MAL-PDT had a delay in appearance of both AKs and SCC.

Prevention of BCC

The search for strategies to prevent BCCs has long been hindered by the lack of an appropriate animal model. BCCs are not observed when the hairless mouse is exposed chronically to UV radiation. The recent availability of a transgenic mouse heterozygous for the PTCH gene provided for the first time an animal model to study prevention strategies for BCC. The PTCH protein, which is a membrane glycoprotein, binds to and inactivates another membrane protein. Mutations in the PTCH or smoothened genes activate the Sonic-Hedgehog (SHH) signalling pathway, which culminates in transformation.

The PTCH$^{+/-}$ mouse develops neoplasms resembling BCC-like tumors when chronically exposed to UV or ionizing radiation. In addition, this mouse model presents several developmental abnormalities found in basal cell nevus syndrome patients, namely polydactyly, medulloblastoma, and jaw cysts.

The current authors recently conducted a study (unpublished) on the ability of PDT with topical methylester ALA to prevent UV-induced BCCs using the PTCH$^{+/-}$ mouse model. In that study, 35 PTCH heterozygous mice were exposed 5 d per

week to UV radiation for a total of 20 weeks. Of these mice, 15 were also treated weekly with topical methylester ALA-PDT. Methylester ALA is cleaved into ALA, which subsequently enters the porphyrin biosynthetic pathway and leads to protoporphyrin IX (PpIX) accumulation. The PTCH$^{+/-}$ mice were sacrificed 8 weeks after the end of UV exposure, and multiple skin biopsies were performed to identify microscopic BCCs. A total of 19 microscopic BCCs were found in nine of the mice exposed to UV radiation only, whereas no BCCs were seen in mice exposed to UV radiation and treated weekly with methylaminolevulinic acid (MAL) PDT. To the current authors' knowledge, this is the first study looking at the ability of large-surface PDT to prevent BCC in PTCH$^{+/-}$ mice. As MAL is transformed into ALA, the current authors believe that large-surface ALA-PDT will also be able to prevent BCCs in this mouse model.

Mechanisms of action of ALA-PDT as a skin cancer preventive modality

The mechanisms of action involved in the ability of ALA-PDT to delay skin cancer appearance are currently under study. The current authors conducted experiments with topical MAL where the photosensitizer was only applied on one half of the back of mice and found that the delay in skin cancer

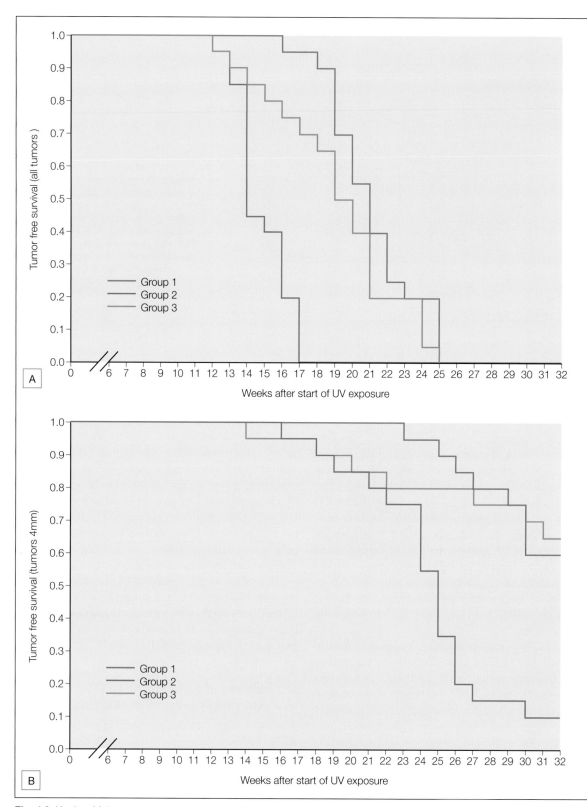

Fig. 4.3 Kaplan–Meier curve showing a delay in all tumors as well as SCC (tumors ≥ 4 mm) induced by topical ALA-PDT in hairless mice. Group 1 was only exposed to UV radiation 5 d per week for 8 weeks. Group 2 was also treated weekly with ALA-PDT, which was started at the same time as UV exposure. Group 3 was exposed to UV radiation for 8 weeks followed by weekly topical ALA-PDT. Reproduced from Liv et al. J Cut Med Surg 8:131;2004 with permission from Springer-Verlag

appearance was only observed on the side where methylaminolevulinate was applied, suggesting a local rather than a systemic effect.

Investigations conducted in the hairless mouse model have shown that chronic UV exposure induces islands of epidermal cells bearing mutations in the p53 gene. This event occurs as early as 17 d after initiation of daily UV exposure and well before any visible lesions are present on mouse skin. Subsequent investigations have shown that patients with chronic sun exposure also exhibit the same type of islands of epidermal cells harbouring p53 mutations, suggesting that these clones of epidermal cells are precursors of visible AKs. Therefore, destruction of these clones by ALA-PDT might prevent the appearance of AKs and eventually the appearance of skin cancer. In a further effort by the current authors to understand the underlying mechanisms of action of ALA-PDT, they recently used immunohistochemistry with a p53 monoclonal antibody to determine whether ALA-PDT sessions would induce a preferential phototoxic reaction in these islands of mutated epidermal cells. Twenty-four hours after ALA-PDT in the hairless mice, the number of keratinocytes showing signs of photo-toxicity from light exposure were not higher on islands of mutated epidermal cells compared to adjacent epidermis, suggesting that these cells are not directly targeted by a phototoxic reaction following ALA-PDT (Fig. 4.4). It is however possible that the cellular photodamage generated by ALA-PDT induces specific toxicity in these islands of mutated epidermal cells by an indirect phenomenon. Other possible mechanisms for skin cancer prevention by ALA-PDT include a cytokine-mediated effect that could either delay tumor growth or reverse UV-induced immunosuppression as well as specific anti-tumoral immune-mediated effects.

Skin Cancer Prevention with PDT in the Clinic

Strictly speaking, the use of ALA-PDT for the treatment of AKs can be considered a skin cancer prevention intervention as AKs are premalignant lesions. However, for the purpose of this chapter prevention of skin cancer with ALA-PDT will be defined as the treatment of skin areas devoid of visible malignant or premalignant lesions with the intention of preventing the appearance of such lesions. At present the use of PDT as a skin cancer preventive modality is still considered experimental. The only approved indication for ALA-PDT in the USA and Canada is the treatment of nonhyper-trophic AKs on the face and scalp.

Despite the lack of official approval, some dermatologists have started to use large-surface ALA-PDT as a skin preventive strategy in their practice. This was done based on the animal studies discussed previously as well as the preliminary safety and efficacy results from studies conducted with large-surface ALA-PDT for treatment of extensive AKs and photoaging.

Patient selection

Patients with only a few AKs are best treated with one or two ALA-PDT sessions, or with another treatment modality such as liquid nitrogen. Patients

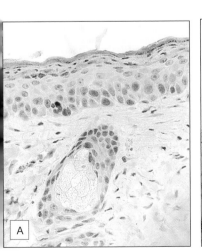
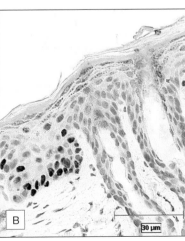

Fig. 4.4 These micrographs are from a hairless mouse exposed weekly to UV radiation and treated once with ALA-PDT. Twenty-four hours post-PDT the photodamage induced by ALA–PDT is mostly located in the upper epidermis (**A**) whereas clusters of cells with mutated p53 (induced by chronic UV exposure) are present in the lower epidermis (**B**)

who can benefit from ALA-PDT for skin cancer prevention include patients: (1) with numerous ill-defined AKs, (2) with frequent new AKs, SCCs or BCCs despite standard treatment, and (3) who are at higher risk of developing skin cancer.

At present ALA-PDT for prevention of skin cancer is mostly used in patients with AKs that are difficult to treat. These are usually either large or confluent AKs or lesions with ill-defined margins. For these patients, large-surface ALA-PDT is performed in order to treat visible lesions as well as microscopic lesions that would eventually develop into AKs. The efficacy of this approach in treating numerous ill-defined AKs has been confirmed in a pilot study. However the long-term prevention of recurrences remains to be studied.

Multiple ALA-PDT sessions can also be used in patients with a history of frequent new AKs or invasive skin cancer despite standard care. Many immunocompetent AK patients will present a complete response following initial therapy, whether with ALA-PDT or another modality, with very few new lesions on subsequent follow-up visits. These patients may be managed with photoprotection and yearly skin examinations. However, some patients will develop numerous new AKs and sometimes even invasive SCC. For these patients, a more aggressive approach might be beneficial. Following treatment of all lesions, either with PDT or another modality, it is possible to perform regular ALA-PDT sessions to try to prevent the appearance of new lesions. The same strategy could be used in patients with basal cell nevus syndrome. Recently Itkin and Gilchrest performed full-face ALA-PDT on two patients with Gorlin's syndrome to decrease the number of new BCCs following treatment.

Multiple ALA-PDT sessions could also be performed in patients without a history of skin cancer but with a very high risk of developing BCC, SCC or AK. These would include patients with genetic disorders that predispose to skin cancer such as basal cell nevus syndrome (Gorlin's syndrome) and xeroderma pigmentosum, as well as organ transplant recipients. The current authors' unpublished study on the prevention of skin cancer in a mouse model for Gorlin's syndrome suggests that multiple PDT sessions can delay photocarcinogenesis if started before the appearance of the first BCC. There is no data yet available for xeroderma pigmentosum (XP). XP patients have an impaired ability to repair DNA, which makes their epidermal cells highly sensitive to transformation following DNA strand breaks induced by UV radiation. As some in vitro studies have suggested that ALA-PDT can be genotoxic, a cautious approach is suggested for XP patients.

Some physicians prefer to wait for studies confirming the efficacy of this preventive therapy before using multiple large-surface ALA-PDT sessions in patients who have never previously presented with malignant or pre-malignant lesions.

ALA-PDT sessions
ALA application

Before large-surface ALA application, a careful skin examination is mandatory to exclude the presence of malignant lesions such as melanoma, lentigo maligna, SCC or BCC. The response of invasive SCC to ALA-PDT has been reported to be disappointing, although some investigators have had success when multiple ALA-PDT sessions are used. The treatment of BCC with MAL is currently approved in several European countries and ALA-PDT has been used with success for the treatment of BCC. However the method has never been standardized and centers often use different protocols, vehicles and/or light sources. The main risk in performing ALA-PDT for BCC or SCC using suboptimal conditions is tumor recurrence. As the initial superficial clinical response is usually very good, these recurrences may arise more deeply and may eventually require extensive surgery. The current authors therefore suggest biopsy of any lesion suspicious of skin cancer before initiating ALA-PDT for skin cancer prevention.

ALA should be applied on all areas where skin prevention is required. Most often this is on the face. The current authors' strategy using the commercially available ALA solution (Levulan) is to first apply ALA on all visible AKs and to let the solution dry. This is followed by a broad application of the solution on the areas to be treated and finally by a second application on all visible AKs. The total volume of ALA solution provided by one commercially available applicator is sufficient to completely cover the face. It is important that care be taken to completely crush both the ALA and the vehicle vials in order to have enough solution available for a full-face application. There are currently no studies available on the influence of the applied hydro-alcoholic solution volume on PpIX synthesis in the skin. As many European dermatologists compound ALA at 5% with good results for the treatment of

AKs and BCCs, a single application of ALA at 20% in the commercially available vehicle should be sufficient. However, this remains to be studied.

After broad-area application, the current authors keep patients in a subdued-light environment (closed ambient lighting in an examination room). Again, studies are not available to confirm if this is necessary. It is probably not essential if light exposure takes place at 1 h after application as little PpIX is generated by the epidermis in the first 30 min after ALA application. Exposure to low-energy output from ambient lighting may even be beneficial in enhancing the efficacy of the ALA-PDT treatment.

Light source and time of light exposure

The Blue-U fluorescent light source is currently the only light source approved for the spot treatment of AKs. In theory any light source providing sufficient output in the spectral range of one of the excitation peaks of PpIX could be used. The current authors favor the use of the Blue-U as two multicenter randomized, controlled studies have defined parameters for good efficacy in the treatment of AKs with this source. Small opaque plastic eyeshields are used to cover the eyes during light exposure. In the current FDA-approved protocol for the treatment of AK with ALA-PDT, light exposure takes place between 14–18 h after ALA application. A recent small pilot study suggested that good efficacy for the treatment of AK can also be obtained when light exposure takes place as early as 1 h after ALA application. The authors of that study did not find a significant difference in clinical response of AK when light exposure took place at either 1 or 3 h after ALA application. The current authors use $10\,J/cm^2$ (the approved light dose for the treatment of AKs) at 1 h after ALA application. Other physicians are using a lower fluence with apparently good results.

In the current authors' experience, inter-patient variability was noted in both the response in AK clearance and the magnitude of the phototoxic reaction following ALA-PDT performed with light exposure at 1 h. For some patients, it seems that 1 h is not enough. Increasing the incubation time to 2 or 3 h on subsequent exposures will induce AK clearance and a mild to moderate phototoxic response. At present it is unknown if the intensity of the phototoxic response present 24 h after ALA-PDT has an influence on the efficacy of the skin preventive strategy. In hairless mice the current authors have shown that ALA-PDT performed using sub-erythematous or erythematous fluences are both efficacious in inducing a delay in skin cancer appearance. In their current approach, effort is made to obtain a mild to moderate erythema on all treated areas of patients at 24 h after light exposure. Further studies will need to be conducted to evaluate the importance of the phototoxic reaction for long-term prevention of skin cancer.

The current authors sometimes use a pulsed-dye laser as a light source (V-Star, Cynosure, Chelmsford, MA) to try to prevent skin cancer development with ALA-PDT. The main advantage of the PDL in their experience is a decrease in pain during treatment. In addition a full-face treatment can be performed in only a few minutes as compared to 16 min 40 s using the Blue-U at $10\,mW/cm^2$. They use the following parameters: 595 nm with a 10 mm spot size at 40 ms pulse duration and subpurpuric fluences of $7–8\,J/cm^2$. A recently published open-label study of the treatment of AKs with PDT performed with ALA and a pulsed-dye laser showed a high clinical response rate using similar settings. Intense pulsed-light sources have also been used for the treatment of AKs with ALA-PDT as the red excitation peaks of PpIX are included in their spectral output.

Number of sessions

Topical ALA-PDT sessions performed on hairless mice weekly, every 2 weeks or every month, have all shown the ability to decrease the appearance of skin cancer. Unfortunately as such studies have not been performed in patients it is not possible to use evidence-based data to determine the ideal frequency for performing preventive ALA-PDT sessions. For some patients, whole-face ALA-PDT as frequently as every 2 weeks may be required to prevent AKs and SCCs (Iltefat Hamzavi, personal communication) whereas others may be treated only once or twice a year. Immunosuppressed patients may require more frequent treatments. These authors' current approach is to first perform large-surface ALA-PDT sessions once or twice a year and then increase treatment frequency should many AKs or SCC lesions develop between treatments.

Side effects

Pain is the most frequent side effect of ALA-PDT. All patients in the pilot study using broad-area PDT at 1 h and more than 90% of patients in the multicenter studies using spot treatment of AK at

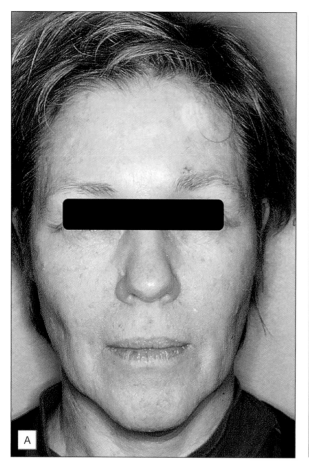
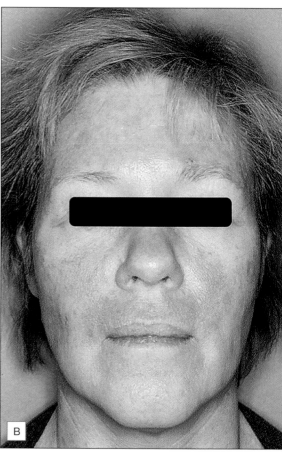

Fig. 4.5 Patient with extensive photodamage and numerous ill-defined AKs before (**A**) and 24 h after (**B**) large-surface ALA-PDT

14–18 h reported pain during light exposure. The pain usually begins shortly after the light source is turned on, increases gradually to reach a plateau, which is often followed by a decrease in pain intensity towards the end of exposure. This pain is believed to be caused by PpIX activation during light exposure and can be easily alleviated by a pause in light exposure. Pain has been reported to be less intense when light exposure takes place at 1 h as compared to 14–18 h. The current authors found that the Smart Cool device sold to be used in conjunction with the Cynosure PDL (Cynosure Chelmsford, MA) provides an excellent method of alleviating pain during light exposure with the Blue-U. Other strategies to manage pain include the use of a fan, spraying of water on the areas that are exposed to light as well as stopping light exposure and applying ice packs. Infiltration with lidocaine can be used if one or two lesions (AKs) are more

painful but this is of limited usefulness when a full face is treated. Some patients also experience post treatment pain, which usually subsides within 24–48 h.

Erythema and edema following large-surface ALA-PDT for skin cancer prevention can be considered a desirable phenomenon. Patients have to be warned that they will undergo a moderate sunburn-like reaction on the exposed area. The intensity of the reaction is highly variable with some patients presenting almost no erythema, while others present severe erythema (Fig. 4.5), sometimes even with focal crusting. This reaction probably depends on the amount of PpIX present in the skin at the time of light exposure.

From a practical standpoint, working with 20% ALA in the hydroalcoholic solution, the main factors that could influence PpIX formation are the time between ALA application and light exposure, the peed of ALA penetration through the stratum corneum barrier and the extent of photodamage. Therefore, care must be taken when modifying the incubation time. For example, a patient who is usually exposed to light 1 h after ALA application can have a much more severe erythematous photo-toxic reaction if light exposure takes place inadvertently for 2 or 3 h on that day.

Care should also be taken when treating patients who are using topical retinoids, alpha hydroxyl acids or other keratolytic agents. These agents may enhance ALA penetration and increase post-treatment erythema and edema. Wood's lamp provides an easy and accessible tool for evaluating PpIX levels in the skin. PpIX exhibits a characteristic pink–red fluorescence when viewed under long-wave UVA and blue light radiation. The human skin is usually devoid of such fluorescence except for follicular (1 mm) dot fluorescence on facial skin that is believed to be of bacterial origin, as well as large red fluorescent areas on psoriasis plaques that are generated by PpIX present in the scales. In the current authors' practice, the skin is always examined 1 h after ALA application with a UVA lamp (Black-Ray long model B-100, UVP, Upland, CA). Red–pink fluorescence is usually absent 1 h after ALA application. In cases where red–pink fluorescence is seen at 1 h, patients have all had at least a moderate phototoxic reaction the day following PDT. Therefore, when PpIX fluorescence is present at 1 h in a new patient, the patient is advised to expect moderate to sometimes severe erythema and edema 24 h after light exposure.

There is always the option to expose only a small skin area for the first treatment if PpIX fluorescence is present at 1 h after ALA application. Sensitivity of a Wood's lamp to detect PpIX fluorescence depends on its exact spectral and power outputs. It is therefore suggested to always use the same Wood's lamp. Patients with extensive sun damage have been observed to often present a more important phototoxic reaction 24 h following PDT. This could be related to higher cellular levels of PpIX accumulated by sun-damaged keratinocytes as the current authors have demonstrated in hairless mice chronically exposed to UV radiation.

Post-PDT erythema usually recedes within 7–10 d. This situation is completely different from what is seen in patients treated with 5-fluorouracil where erythema often persists for weeks and sometimes months after therapy. The intensity of the reaction is not as severe as what is usually seen when imiquimod is used in patients with AKs and extensive sun damage. The erythema generated by ALA-PDT is very similar to a sunburn and the current authors have never seen the purpura-like reaction that can sometimes be observed in imiquimod-treated patients.

All patients should be warned about potential phototoxic reactions following sun exposure, especially when facial treatments are performed. This is definitely important when light exposure takes place at 1 h after ALA application as skin peak PpIX levels have not yet reached maximum intensity and new PpIX is synthesized after light exposure. Patients should be advised to avoid spending time outdoors for 2 d after ALA application. They should also avoid intense broad-spectrum light such as dental or operating room lights on areas where ALA was applied. Patients should be instructed that current sunscreens do not protect well against visible light.

Hyperpigmentation and hypopigmentation can occur after ALA-PDT. This is usually not seen in patients with phototype II–III when the treatment is performed on the face. The risks are higher with the treatment of extrafacial regions, especially the legs. The current authors have never seen scarring following large-surface ALA-PDT for skin cancer prevention. Scarring is sometimes seen after the treatment of tumors with ALA-PDT but it could be argued that it arises from previous destruction of normal tissue by the original tumoral process.

Can multiple ALA-PDT sessions induce the appearance of skin cancer? There has been one case report of a malignant melanoma developing on the scalp of a patient who had previously received ALA-PDT for AKs and superficial SCC. Some in vitro studies have also suggested that ALA could be genotoxic on cell lines. In order to evaluate the carcinogenic potential of ALA-PDT, these authors have treated a group of 20 hairless mice weekly with ALA-PDT (no UV exposure) for a total of 10 months and failed to observe a single tumor. Although ALA-PDT is reminiscent of PUVA (Psoralen-UVA) therapy, there are important differences. Whereas psoralens are present in the nucleus and induce the formation of covalent bonds with DNA upon UV activation, PpIX localizes to the cytoplasm and is believed to react mostly with intracellular membranes. These differences as well as animal studies conducted so far do not point towards an increased risk of skin cancer following ALA-PDT.

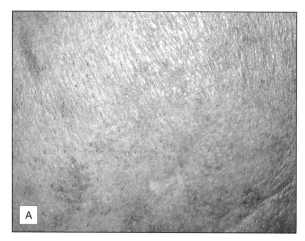

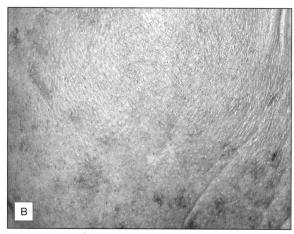

Fig. 4.6 Patient with AKs before (**A**) and after (**B**) large-surface ALA-PDT

Benefits

Large-surface ALA-PDT performed at 1 h after ALA application has been shown to induce a good complete response rate in patients with multiple AKs (Fig. 4.6). These authors have also had good success with the treatment of AKs using this strategy. Unfortunately, human data on the prevention of skin cancer with repeated large-surface ALA-PDT sessions is not currently available. The pilot study of full-face ALA-PDT performed in patients with multiple AKs has also shown improvement in signs of photoaging, which is an additional benefit for patients.

Future directions

Long-term clinical studies are definitely needed to assess the efficacy of ALA-PDT as a skin cancer prevention modality. Separate studies should be performed for different populations such as patients with a history of multiple AKs and/or SCC, immunosuppressed patients and Gorlin's syndrome patients. These studies should aim at assessing the ability of multiple ALA–PDT sessions in preventing skin cancer as well as to study the influence of different parameters such as light fluence, ALA incubation time, and frequency of treatments. Such a study is currently underway with methylaminolevulinate. It is a randomized contralateral controlled study of the ability of methylaminolevulinate-PDT to prevent new tumors in immunosuppressed patients. A total of eight large-surface PDT sessions are planned over a period of 15 months. In addition, DUSA Pharmaceuticals is currently planning a multicenter split face study to look at comparing the efficacy of multiple ALA-PDT sessions in photoaging to light alone. As a secondary efficacy measure the number of new AKs appearing on treated sites during the trial will be monitored. Results of these trials could provide clinical evidence of the ability of large-surface PDT to prevent skin cancer

Conclusion

Multiple large-surface ALA-PDT sessions have been shown to delay the induction of AKs, SCCs, as well as BCCs, in mice. A recent pilot study has shown that large-surface ALA-PDT, with a short incubation time, is safe and can induce rapid clearing of AKs. Based on these findings, repetitive large-surface ALA-PDT is currently used by many physicians in order to try to prevent skin cancer. Future studies are needed to confirm and measure the efficacy of multiple ALA-PDT sessions in preventing skin cancer in different patient populations.

Further Reading

Alexiades-Armenakas MR, Geronemus RG 2003 Laser-mediated photodynamic therapy of actinic keratoses. Archives of Dermatology 139(10):1313–1320

Aszterbaum M, Epstein J, Oro A et al 1999 Ultraviolet and ionizing radiation enhance the growth of BCCs and trichoblastomas in patched heterozygous knockout mice. Nature Medicine 5(11):1285–1291

Avram DK, Goldman MP 2004 Effectiveness and safety of ALA-IPL in treating actinic keratoses and photodamage. Journal of Drugs in Dermatology 3(suppl):S36–S39

Bissonnette R, Bergeron A, Liu Y 2004 Large surface photodynamic therapy with aminolevulinic acid: treatment of actinic keratoses and beyond. Journal of Drugs in Dermatology 3:S26–S31

de Gruijl FR, Forbes PD 1995 UV-induced skin cancer in a hairless mouse model. Bioessays 17(7):651–660

Duffield-Lillico AJ, Slate EH, Reid ME et al 2003 Nutritional prevention of cancer study group. Selenium supplementation and secondary prevention of nonmelanoma skin cancer in a randomized trial. Journal of the National Cancer Institute 95(19):1477–1481

Fung TT, Spiegelman D, Egan KM et al 2003 Vitamin and carotenoid intake and risk of squamous cell carcinoma of the skin. International Journal of Cancer 103(1):110–115

Goldman MP, Atkin DH 2003 ALA/PDT in the treatment of actinic keratosis: Spot vs. confluent therapy. Journal of Cosmetic Laser Therapy 5:107–110

Housman TS, Feldman SR, Williford PM et al 2003 Skin cancer is among the most costly of all cancers to treat for the Medicare population. Journal of the American Academy of Dermatology 48(3):425–429

Itkin A, Gilchrest BA 2004 delta-Aminolevulinic acid ahD blue light photodynamic therapy for treatment of multiple basal cell carcinoma in two patients with nevoid basal cell carcinoma. Dermatology Surgery 30(7):1054–1061

Kuchide M, Tokuda H, Takayasu J et al 2003 Cancer chemopreventive effects of oral feeding alpha-tocopherol on ultraviolet light B induced photocarcinogenesis of hairless mouse. Cancer Letters 196(2):169–177

Levine N, Moon TE, Cartmel B et al l997 Trial of retinol and isotretinoin in skin cancer prevention: a randomized, double-blind, controlled trial. Cancer Epidemiology, Biomarkers and Prevention 6(11):957–961

Piacquadio DJ, Chen DM, Farber HF et al 2004 Photodynamic therapy with aminolevulinic acid topical solution and visible blue light in the treatment of multiple actinic keratoses of the face and scalp: investigator-blinded, phase 3, multicenter trials. Archives of Dermatology 140(1):41–46

Sharfaei S, Juzenas P, Moon J et al 2002 Weekly topical application of methyl aminolevulinate followed by light exposure delays the appearance of UV-induced skin tumours in mice. Archives of Dermatology Research 294:237–242

Sharfaei S, Viau G, Lui H et al 2001 Systemic photodynamic therapy with aminolevulinic acid delays the appearance of ultraviolet-induced skin tumours in mice. British Journal of Dermatology 144(6):1207–1214

Stender IM, Beck-Thomsen N, Poulsen T et al 1997 Photodynamic therapy with topical delta-aminolevulinic acid delays UV photo-cardinogenesis in hairless mice. Photochemistry and Photobiology 66:493–496

Touma D, Yaar M, Whitehead S et al 2004 A trial of short incubation, broad-area photodynamic therapy for facial actinic keratoses and diffuse photodamage. Archives of Dermatology 140(1):33–40

5

Treatment of Skin Cancer

Sigrid Karrer, Rolf-Markus Szeimies

Introduction

The problem being treated

Photodynamic therapy (PDT) is a treatment modality with unique properties that make it an appealing procedure for the treatment of nonmelanoma skin cancer. Topical PDT using 5-aminolevulinic acid (ALA) or the methyl ester of 5-aminolevulinic acid (MAL) is based on the photosensitization of the target tissue by ALA- or MAL-induced porphyrins and subsequent irradiation with red light inducing cell death in a dose-dependent manner via generation of reactive oxygen species.

Up to now topical ALA-PDT has been successfully used for the management of precancerous lesions, including actinic keratoses (AKs) and Bowen's disease (see Ch. 3) and superficial, non-melanoma skin tumors, mainly basal cell carcinoma (BCC) and early stages of squamous cell carcinoma (SCC). The efficacy of MAL-PDT in the treatment of patients with AKs and superficial or nodular BCCs has been investigated in several phase II and III clinical trials. Currently in Europe, Australia and New Zealand MAL (Metvix, Photocure AS, Norway, and Galderma SA, France) is approved for the photodynamic treatment of superficial and nodular BCCs and AKs in combination with red light. In the USA, MAL has been recently (July 2004) approved for the treatment of AK in combination with red light. ALA (Levulan Kerastick, DUSA, USA) has been approved since 2000 in the USA for PDT of AKs in combination with blue light.

Other potential indications for topical ALA-PDT are cutaneous T-cell lymphoma, metastatic breast carcinoma, and metastasis from malignant melanoma, but for these indications clinical results have been either disappointing or the evidence from the literature is weak. Therefore, in this chapter only the two established indications for topical PDT of skin tumors, BCC and early incipient SCC, will be discussed in detail.

SCC is a malignant, potentially metastasizing tumor arising from the keratinocytes of the epidermis. Cumulative excessive lifetime exposure to sunlight is the major cause of SCC. In situ forms of SCC are AKs or Bowen's disease. SCC begins when atypical keratinocytes break through the basement membrane and begin to invade the dermis. Surgery or radiotherapy are the most common approaches to treat invasive SCC. However, for early invasive SCC, topical ALA-PDT may also be effective and offer pleasing cosmetic results.

BCC is a malignant, but exceedingly rarely metastasizing tumor of the skin that arises from basal cells in the epidermis. It is the most common malignant tumor of the skin in white races. BCCs are usually located in sun-exposed areas of the skin: the face, head and neck region, trunk and upper extremities (Table 5.1). Treatment of BCC depends on tumor size, location and clinical type (Fig. 5.1).

Nodular BCCs have well-defined borders and grow vertically. Owing to the greater thickness of

Localization of BCCs		
Region	(%)	(%)
Head, neck		85
Nose	30	
Face	21	
Front	15	
Ear	7	
Trunk, extremities		15

Table 5.1 Localization of BCCs (Adapted from A Kopf 1979 Journal of Dermatology)

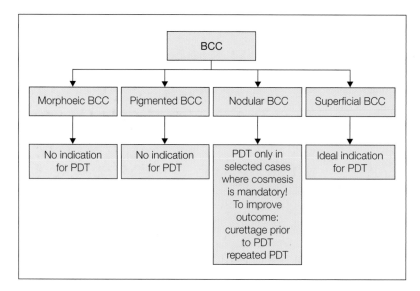

Fig. 5.1 Basal cell carcinoma (BCC): indication for topical PDT

the tumor, nodular BCCs should be preferentially treated by surgery. Pigmented BCCs do not allow an optimal penetration of the light and are therefore not an indication for PDT. Morpheaform BCCs grow with diffuse borders and are often larger than expected. Therefore, the treatment of morpheaform BCC should be surgical, with preference of Mohs micrographic surgery with pathological control of excision margins (Fig. 5.2). Superficial BCCs usually occur on the trunk and are often multiple. Several modalities exist for the treatment of superficial BCC, and these include cryotherapy, curettage and cautery, cytotoxic agents, radiotherapy and excisional surgery. Surgery may be complicated by obvious scars and the requirement for complex reconstruction while cryotherapy or topical chemotherapy may require multiple treatments and may result in poor cosmetic results or recurrence of the tumor. Therefore, topical PDT offers a tissue-sparing modality with excellent cosmesis. Topical PDT with ALA or MAL in patients with superficial BCC achieves clearance rates of up to 100% following a single treatment.

The aim of curative PDT of skin tumors is the complete destruction of the tumor. Owing to the limited penetration of red light into tissue, the thickness of tumors should not exceed 2–3 mm when surface illumination is used. When treating nodular BCCs by single ALA-PDT, the cure rate is rather low, with an average cure rate below 50%. In order to ameliorate poor outcome after PDT of thicker BCC lesions, ALA-PDT has been performed

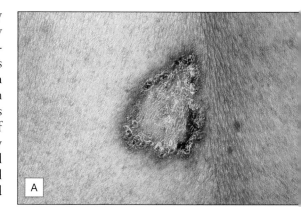

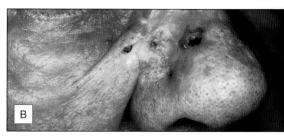

Fig. 5.2 (A) Pigmented BCC. (B) Morphoeic BCC. Both histological subtypes of BCC are not suitable for topical ALA-PDT

by Thissen 3 weeks after prior debulking of the tumor. The former tumor areas were excised 3 months later and histopathologically evaluated for residual tumor. Clinically and histologically, a complete response was observed in 92% of the treated lesions.

ALA-PDT can also be used for adjuvant therapy in combination with Mohs surgery, as reported recently by Kuijpers et al. In four patients who underwent Mohs micrographic surgery for extensive BCC, first the central infiltrating tumor part was excised. After re-epithelialization, ALA-PDT of the surrounding tumor rims (2–5 cm) bearing remaining superficial tumor parts was performed. This led to a complete remission of the tumors with excellent clinical and cosmetic results (follow-up period 27 months).

Remission rates after ALA-PDT can be probably improved by also using other modified treatment modalities, such as repeated treatments or addition of penetration enhancers like dimethyl sulfoxide (DMSO) or ethylenediamine tetra-acetic acid (EDTA).

The methods of PDT are continuously advancing. So far the proven advantages of PDT include comparable clinical outcome to standard treatments, the simultaneous treatment of multiple tumors and incipient lesions, relatively short healing times, tumor control in immunocompromised patients (i.e. transplant recipients), good patient tolerance and excellent cosmesis.

Patient Selection

Except for exclusion of patients with known history of porphyries or allergic reactions to active ingredients of the applied sensitizers, no severe contraindications for MAL/ALA-PDT are known. MAL/ALA-PDT should be considered in particular for patients who have extensive, widespread or multiple low-risk superficial lesions, as those in nevoid BCC syndrome. Also, immunosuppressed patients after organ transplantation, who often suffer from multiple lesions, are good candidates for PDT. Elderly patients who would require hospitalization for surgery or in whom radiation therapy would involve multiple daily treatment sessions benefit from PDT, since PDT is usually performed on an outpatient basis, is not invasive and does not require local anesthesia (see Box 5.1).

PDT can be repeated several times and even in areas with prior exposure to ionizing irradiation PDT is possible.

Expected Benefits

ALA-PDT for BCC has been studied in the past years extensively in a variety of surveys (Table 5.2). The weighted average of complete clearance rates, after follow-up periods varying between 3 and 36 months, was 87% in 12 studies treating 826 superficial BCCs and 53% in 208 nodular BCCs as reviewed by Peng. Available compiled data by Zeitouni from other trials have shown an average of 87% for superficial BCCs, and 48% for nodular BCCs (Figs 5.3–5.5).

MAL-PDT for BCC achieves clearance rates of around 80% for nodular (debulking prior to PDT) and superficial BCC after two PDT sessions administered 7 d apart (Table 5.3).

In a prospective phase III trial comparing ALA-PDT with cryosurgery, Wang et al included 88 superficial and nodular BCCs. A 20% ALA/water-in-oil cream was applied for 6 h under an occlusive dressing, followed by irradiation with a laser at 635 nm (80 mW/cm², 60 J/cm²). In the cryosurgery arm, lesions were treated with liquid nitrogen employing the open spray technique using two freeze–thaw cycles for 25–30 s each time. After 3 months, punch biopsies were performed and revealed a recurrence rate of 25% in the PDT group and 15% in the cryosurgery group. However, the clinical recurrence rates were only 5% for ALA-PDT and 13% for cryosurgery. Besides a better cosmetic outcome, the healing time was also shorter in the PDT-treated group.

Tumor thickness is a determinant of the response of BCC to ALA-PDT. A clearance rate of 100% was achieved by Morton with an ALA application time of 6 h for BCCs < 2 mm in thickness.

Although cure rates of up to 100% after PDT of superficial BCC have been shown in several studies, some studies have shown a decrease of the cure rate to 50–60% after long-term follow up. The current

Summary of results of clinical studies using topical ALA-PDT for the treatment of BCC				
Study	**Indication / procedure**	**No. of lesions**	**Complete remission (%)**	**Follow up**
Fink-Puches 1998	Superficial BCC	95	50	36 months
Morton 1998	Superficial BCC < 2 mm thickness, 6 h incubation	26	100	6–16 months
Thissen 2000	Nodular BCCs (debulking 3 weeks prior to PDT)	24	92	3 months (histological control)
Haller 2000	Superficial BCC (double treatment within 7 d)	26	96	15–45 months
Wang 2001	Superficial and nodular BCC	44	75 (histologically) 95 (clinically)	3 months (histological control)
Varma 2001	Superficial BCC	61	82	12 months
Clark 2003	Superficial BCC	87	97	12 months

Table 5.2 Summary of results of clinical studies using topical ALA-PDT for the treatment of BCC

authors observed recurrences of BCC even after 3 years following ALA-PDT in single patients. Therefore, a long-term follow-up of at least 12 months and preferably 3 years after PDT is mandatory for early detection of recurrent tumors. In the case of tumor recurrence, the current authors would recommend to re-treatment by surgery since this therapy allows histological examination.

There are few studies on ALA-PDT of SCC. Most studies showed recurrence rates of greater than 50%. Owing to the high recurrence rates and the metastatic potential of SCC, PDT should be reserved for patients with initial SCC in whom surgery is strongly contraindicated or for immuno-suppressed patients requiring field reduction of numerous, early, incipient, superficial SCCs prior to more targeted surgical treatment of more invasive, larger SCCs that persist.

Besides clinical efficacy, cost effectiveness is an important aspect of determining the overall benefit of PDT. Cost analysis indicates that with relatively low costs for permanent equipment, topical ALA-PDT is comparable in cost with other therapies when morbidity costs of standard treatments are included, and PDT is more economical in patients with multiple tumors who can be treated in a single PDT session. A list of possible complications of ALA-PDT is provided in Table 5.4.

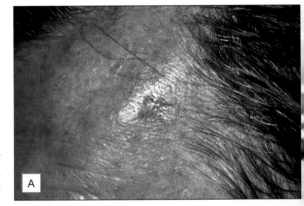

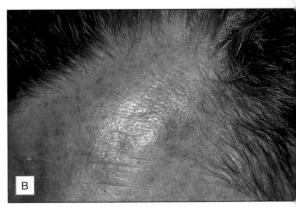

Fig. 5.3 (**A**) 65-year-old man with superficial BCC on left forehead prior to ALA-PDT. (**B**) 3 months after single course of PDT with excellent clinical result – only presence of slight erythema

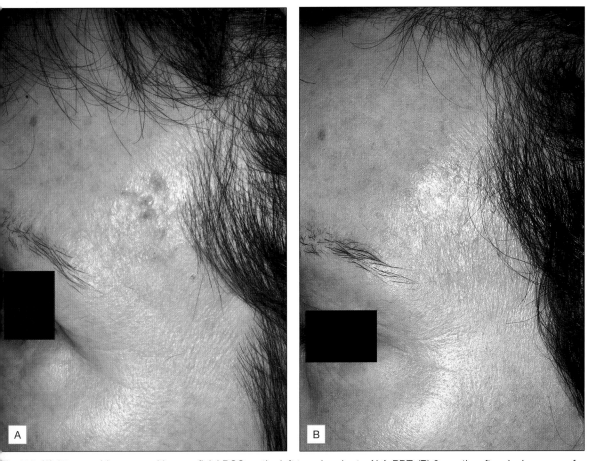

Fig. 5.4 (A) 37-year-old woman with superficial BCC on the left temple prior to ALA-PDT. **(B)** 6 months after single course of PDT: complete clearance and excellent cosmetic result

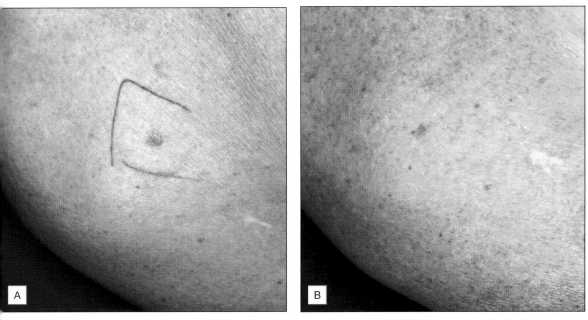

Fig. 5.5 (A) 71-year-old man with superficial BCC on the right shoulder prior to ALA-PDT. **(B)** 6 months after single course of PDT: excellent clinical result

Summary of results of clinical studies using topical MAL-PDT for the treatment of BCC				
Study	Indication / procedure	No. of lesions	Complete remission (%)	Follow up
Soler 2001	Nodular and superficial BCCs (debulking of nodular BCCs, double treatment within 7 d)	350	79	35 months
Horn 2003	Nodular and superficial BCCs (double treatment within 7 d, nonresponders retreated after 3 months)	123	82	24 months
Rhodes 2004	Nodular BCCs (double treatment within 7 d, nonresponders retreated after 3 months)	53	83	24 months

Table 5.3 Summary of results of clinical studies using topical MAL-PDT for the treatment of BCC

Side effects of ALA-PDT	
Frequency	Possible side effects of ALA-PDT
Usually	Stinging or burning sensation during irradiation Localized erythema and edema after irradiation Crusting and dry necrosis of tumor
Occasionally	Stinging or burning for some hours after irradiation
Rarely	Minor scarring Pigmentary changes (usually resolve) Alopecia in the treatment area

Table 5.4 Side effects of ALA-PDT

Overview of Treatment Strategy

Treatment approach

Patients with superficial nonmelanoma skin tumors, mainly superficial BCC and in selected cases initial SCC, are eligible for ALA-PDT. The advantages and disadvantages of the different treatment modalities for superficial BCC are summarized in Table 5.5.

Major determinants

Patient interviews

In order to identify the best therapeutic option for the patient, it is of utmost importance to take a very careful history of the patient. The patient should be asked the following questions:

1. Do you suffer from porphyria or do you know about a specific allergy against active ingredients of the 5-aminolevulinic acid or methyl amino-levulinate preparation? *(Reason: to exclude possible risk of induction of porphyria by topical administration of 5-ALA or MAL)*
2. Do you take anticoagulants or aspirin? *(Reason: to exclude possible bleeding in case of lesion preparation/curettage before PDT; anticoagulation itself is no contraindication for PDT)*
3. Do you take antioxidants, which might interfere with the photodynamic reaction? *(Reason: to minimize the risk of presence of high levels of antioxidants [vitamin C, E etc.], which perhaps quench the photodynamic reaction)*
4. Do you take nonsteroidal anti-inflammatory drugs. *(Reason: to minimize the risk of presence of high levels of suppressors of the arachidonic pathway which is vital for the inflammatory reaction that contributes to the direct toxic effect of the induction of reactive oxygen species [ROS])*
5. Do you take other photosensitizing drugs such as antimalarials, diuretics, antibiotics etc.? *(Reason: to minimize the risk of overintensity of the phototoxic effect)*
6. Do you take cytostatic drugs such as hydroxyurea, azathioprine or others? *(Reason: to minimize the risk of prolonged healing/re-epithelialization after PDT)*

Treatment techniques

Patients

For patients with a clinical diagnosis of superficial BCC, there are several efficient alternative treatments for therapy of single lesions, including cryotherapy, curettage or surgery. For therapy of multiple superficial BCCs, PDT is a first-line modality (e.g. in basal cell nevus syndrome, immunosuppressed patients after organ transplantation).

Advantages and disadvantages of different treatment options for superficial BCC		
Treatment	**Advantages**	**Disadvantages**
Topical ALA-PDT	Excellent cosmesis Noninvasive Safe Tumor selectivity Simultaneous treatment of multiple tumors Short healing time Cost effective	Pain during PDT Time consuming No histology
Curettage	Cheap and easy to perform Histology	Local anesthesia Scarring Recurrence rate
Cryotherapy	Cheap and fast to perform	Pain during treatment Blistering Delayed wound healing Scarring Hypopigmentation Skin atrophy No histology
Surgery (simple excision)	Safe Histology	Invasive Local anesthesia Scarring

Table 5.5 Advantages and disadvantages of different treatment options for superficial BCC

PDT may also be used in patients with a histological or clinical diagnosis of nodular BCC, if other established treatment modalities are contraindicated, and patients with a histological diagnosis of early or incipient SCC, if other established treatment modalities are contraindicated.

Equipment

PDT is a two-step procedure. For application of the drug, standard material-like bandages or occlusive dressings are necessary. For large tumors or extensive hyperkeratosis, pre-PDT debulking with a ring curette or scalpel is required (Figs 5.6–10).

For the second step, a specific light source is necessary.

Light sources

For irradiation of skin cancer, most often incoherent light sources are used, and these are typically lamps (PDT 1200L, Waldmann Medizintechnik, Germany) or light-emitting diodes (LEDs) (Aktilite, Galderma or Omnilux, Waldmann/Phototherapeutics Ltd., UK), which match the absorption maxima of the 5-ALA- or MAL-induced porphyrins.

Small areas or single lesions can also be efficiently illuminated with different lasers (e.g. argon-ion pumped-dye lasers at 630 nm, gold vapor lasers at 628 nm, diode lasers) as long as they match the specific absorption maximum of the photosensitizer used. However, the costs of purchase and maintenance of laser systems is greater than for incoherent light sources.

For tissue destruction using ALA-PDT, red light (580–700 nm) – of 120–180 J/cm^2 (100–200 mW/cm^2) – may be chosen. For the more narrow emission spectra of the LED systems (bandwidth approximately 30 nm), the fluence values are significantly lower (37–50 J/cm^2). Therefore, for MAL-PDT using the Aktilite LED system, a light dose of 37 J/cm^2 is recommended both for AK and BCC. In any case, the light intensity should not exceed 200 mW/cm^2 to avoid hyperthermic effects. During illumination, both the patient and clinic staff should be wearing protective goggles in order to avoid the risk of eye damage.

In a comparative trial it was shown that light at shorter wavelengths is less effective in the treatment of Bowen's disease at a theoretically equivalent dose; therefore only the use of red light is recommended for PDT of skin tumors in order to maximize tissue penetration.

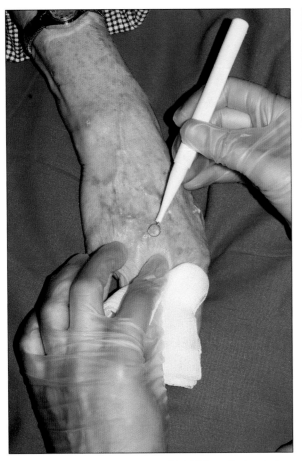

Fig. 5.6 74-year-old patient with initial SCC on the back of the hands. Curettage of the hyperkeratotic parts of the tumor with a Stiefel curette

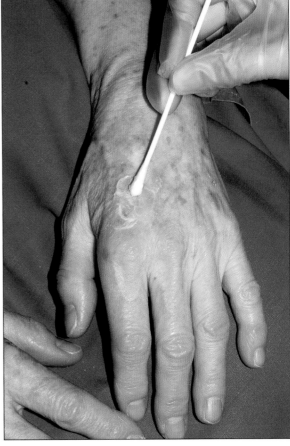

Fig. 5.7 Application of 5-ALA cream (20% ALA in unguentum emulsificans). Either a swab or a wooden spatula can be used for application. Drug should be applied with 1 mm thickness at least with an 0.5–1 cm overlap

Photosensitizer

In the USA the Levulan Kerastick (DUSA, USA), containing 5-ALA hydrochloride is approved for photodynamic treatment of AKs in combination with blue light. In Europe, Australia and New Zealand, MAL (Metvix, Photocure AS, Norway, and Galderma SA, France) is approved for the photodynamic treatment of superficial and nodular BCC and AKs in combination with red light (in the USA, it is so far only approved for AKs). MAL is more lipophilic than ALA and might therefore result in an increased tumor penetration after topical application.

For the treatment of skin tumors, usually ALA as hydrochloride (Crawford Pharmaceuticals, UK; photonamic GmbH, Germany) is applied in custom-made formulations, either oil-in-water emulsions or gels, at a concentration of 20%. However, no comparative data on different formulations exist. ALA preparations are mostly applied to the lesions under occlusion and in addition to a light protecting dressing or clothing for 4–6 h prior to irradiation.

Since June 2001 MAL is available as an approved drug (Metvix). For the MAL ointment, a shorter incubation time of 3 h is sufficient due to preferential uptake and higher selectivity. The entire area is then covered with an occlusive foil to allow for better penetration.

Enhancement of ALA-PDT has been studied using the penetration enhancer DMSO and the iron chelators desferrioxamine and EDTA, but there are no randomized comparison data.

Treatment algorithm

1. Check patient eligibility for MAL/ALA-PDT:
   - Check indication (if necessary perform a biopsy to prove the diagnosis)

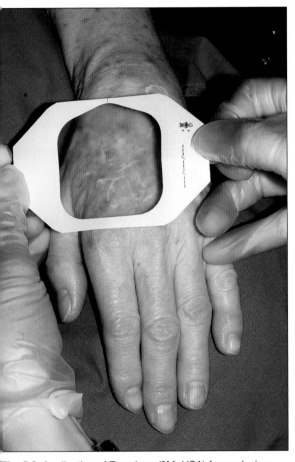

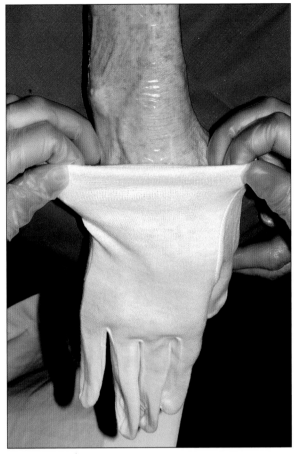

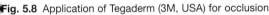

Fig. 5.8 Application of Tegaderm (3M, USA) for occlusion

Fig. 5.9 Use of gloves for light protection. In case of lesions in the face, aluminium foil or simply a hat or cap can be used. Direct contact of aluminium foil with ALA-preparation should be avoided due to the acidity of this preparation

- Check exclusion criteria: pregnancy, allergy to components of the MAL/ALA preparation, porphyria, etc.
- Obtain written informed consent
- Obtain exact documentation of the localization and size of the lesion (photodocumentation prior to therapy might be suitable)

2. Treatment:
- Select the area to be treated
- Check whether crusts or prominent tumor parts are present which might be removed prior to PDT procedure (Fig. 5.6)
- Apply the 20% ALA formulation or the MAL preparation (1 mm thick) to the lesion with little overlap (about 0.5–1 cm) to the surrounding tissue (Fig. 5.7)
- Cover the entire area with an occlusive foil to allow better penetration (Fig. 5.8)

- Then cover the incubated area also with a light protecting dressing or clothing to avoid photobleaching of the induced porphyrins (Fig. 5.9)
- Advise the patient to come back in 3 h (when MAL is applied) or 4–6 h (when ALA is applied)
- Remove the dressing and emulsion after 3 h (for MAL) or 4–6 h (for ALA) of incubation
- Place the lamp/laser within the right distance from the lesion (Fig. 5.10)
- Irradiate with the irradiation parameters advised for the specific illumination system
- After irradiation cover the lesion to avoid exposure to sunlight
- Tell the patient that there will be crusting of the lesion after 2–3 d following PDT, which will resolve within the next 2 weeks
- Tell the patient to come back if infection of the treated area or any other problem occurs

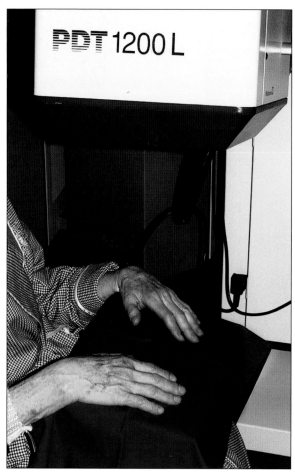

Fig. 5.10 Illumination with incoherent light source after an incubation period of 6 h (Waldmann PDT 1200 L, Waldmann Medizintechnik, Villingen-Schwenningen, Germany)

- No specific post-PDT treatment is required besides avoidance of the sun/sun protection with sunscreens for the next 4–6 weeks
- Careful follow up is mandatory for early detection of recurrence, and recommended intervals are: 4 weeks after PDT, 3 months after PDT, 6 months after PDT, 12 months after PDT, 18 months after PDT, 24 months after PDT and 36 months after PDT
- If thicker tumors (> 3mm) are treated with ALA-PDT, a second treatment session (3–5 weeks apart) is recommended to improve the therapeutic outcome. For MAL-PDT, a second treatment after 7 d is routinely recommended for all tumors treated.

With red light, superficial lesions can be treated in a single session as described earlier. However, thicker lesions can be treated repeatedly with the same parameters starting 3–5 weeks after the first PDT session. Efficacy of PDT in thicker lesions can also be improved by tissue preparation (debulking) prior to PDT. For tissue preparation, a slight curettage without major bleeding is sufficient.

Irradiation should be performed preferentially with red light due to the likelihood of deeper tissue penetration. Irradiation with blue or green light for skin cancer is contraindicated.

The advantages of PDT as compared to surgery or cryotherapy are the good cosmetic results and good tolerability despite a certain discomfort, in particular when larger areas are treated. Further, large areas can be treated in one session. In an overwhelming majority of patients treated for oncologic indications, PDT is very well accepted.

Troubleshooting
Side effects, complications, and alternative approaches

The well-known stinging or burning sensation during topical PDT is usually well tolerated when small areas are treated. However, in case of larger areas (mostly in severely sun-damaged skin) significant discomfort can make analgesia with metamizole or piritramide, or even general or local anesthesia, necessary. Pain perception can also be alleviated by a fan, cold air stream or by pouring water onto the treated area during the illumination procedure. Application of a tetracaine gel 1 h pre-irradiation did not significantly reduce pain during and after PDT in a randomized, double-blind, placebo-controlled study by Holmes. Application of a eutectic mixture of prilocaine/lidocaine (EMLA) should be avoided due to the high pH of this preparation, which might interfere with the acidity of the ALA preparation, leading to a chemical inactivation of the photosensitizer. In addition, topically applied anesthetics also induce local vasoconstriction, which interferes with the generation of sufficient amounts of ROS. Stinging pain and a burning sensation are usually restricted to the time span of illumination and a few hours thereafter.

After light exposure, for several days, localized erythema and edema in the treated area is usually seen, and is followed by a dry necrosis sharply restricted to the tumor. After 10–21 d, formed crusts come off and complete re-epithelialization is observed. During this phase, most patients report only slight discomfort.

The cosmetic outcome of the completely responding lesions is good or very good in most patients. In about 2%, minor scarring occurs, and also uncommon (2%) are pigmentary changes. Some patients experience a temporary pigmentary change with a residual erythematous hue. Irreversible alopecia has not yet been observed in the vast majority of the treated patients; however, due to the concomitant sensitization of the pilosebaceous units, this potential effect should be taken into account. For a list of possible complications of ALA-PDT, see Table 5.4.

When treating invasive tumors, for example, invasive SCC, the lack of histological control and the limited depth of tissue penetration of a single topical PDT treatment must be borne in mind. Therefore, usually only superficial lesions should be treated by PDT and regular follow up is needed to recognize recurrence of the tumor.

Advanced Topics: Treatment Tips for Experienced Practitioners

To improve treatment results, several studies have tried various modifications of the treatment protocol (Tables 5.6, 5.7). Several workers proposed double or even multiple ALA-PDT treatments to improve therapy outcome. In contrast to ALA-PDT, topical PDT with MAL is routinely performed twice within 7 d.

Protocol for topical ALA-PDT of nonmelanoma skin cancer	
Photosensitizer	20% ALA in water in oil emulsion
Lesion preparation	Debulking of exophytic tumor parts or hyperkeratotic crusts using a curette or scalpel
Application	Topical application with little overlap (about 1 cm) to the surrounding tissue, occlusive and light-impermeable dressing
Incubation time	4–6 h
Light source	Red light from an incoherent lamp or laser emitting 635 nm
Irradiation parameters	Light intensity 100–180 mW/cm^2 Light dose 120–180 J/cm^2
Frequency of treatment	Usually single treatment, for larger or thicker tumors repeated treatments (not established)

Table 5.6 Protocol for topical ALA-PDT of nonmelanoma skin cancer

Protocol for topical MAL (Metvix)-PDT of BCC	
Photosensitizer	MAL 160 mg/g topical cream (Metvix)
Lesion preparation	Debulking of exophytic tumor parts or hyperkeratotic crusts using a curette or scalpel
Application	Topical application (1 mm thick, with 0.5–1 cm overlap to the surrounding tissue), adhesive occlusive dressing
Incubation time	3 h
Light source	Red light from an incoherent lamp or LED (light-emitting diode)
Irradiation parameters	Light intensity < 200 mW/cm^2 For lamp: light dose 120–180 J/cm^2 For LED: light dose 37 J/cm^2
Frequency of treatment	Routinely two sessions 1 week apart, repeated if required at 3-month follow up

Table 5.7 Protocol for topical MAL (Metvix)-PDT of BCC

For lesions < 1 cm in diameter, Fritsch et al reported 60%, 80% and 100% recurrence-free CR rates with, respectively 1, 2 and 3 treatments (follow up 12–24 months). In his study the treatments were given at 1-month intervals until CR was achieved. Similarly, Calzavara-Pinton and co-workers repeated ALA-PDT every alternate day (up to a maximum of three treatments) until no tumor was apparent, and achieved 100% CR rate at 30 d, with a recurrence rate of 13% over a follow-up period of 24–36 months. Haller et al chose a 7-day interval between initial and second treatment to provide time for maximum photodynamic damage to develop and for some healing to occur between treatments. With a routine double treatment they achieved a CR of 96% after a median follow-up of 27 months.

However, the optimal timing of repeated treatments remains unknown. Whether it is preferable to observe patients regularly and only re-treat when necessary, or to give a standardized double treatment to all patients is still an open question. Using a routine double treatment would result in about 50% of patients receiving a second PDT that would not have otherwise been required.

Further Reading

Calzavara-Pinton PG 1995 Repetitive photodynamic therapy with topical delta-aminolevulinic acid as an appropriate approach to the routine treatment of superficial non-melanoma skin tumors. Journal of Photochemistry and Photobiology 29:53–57

Clark C, Bryden A, Dawe R et al 2003 Topical 5-aminolaevulinic acid photodynamic therapy for cutaneous lesions: outcome and comparison of light sources. Photodermatology, Photoimmunology and Photomedicine 19:134–141

Foley P 2003 Clinical efficacy of methyl aminolevulinate (Metvix) photodynamic therapy. Journal of Dermatological Treatment 14(suppl 3):15–22

Fritsch C, Goerz G, Ruzicka T 1998 Photodynamic therapy in dermatology. Archives in Dermatology 134:207–214

Guillen C, Sanmartin O, Escudero A et al 2000 Photodynamic therapy for in situ squamous cell carcinoma on chronic radiation dermatitis after photosensitization with 5-aminolevulinic acid. Journal of the European Academy of Dermatology 14:298–300

Haller JC, Cairnduff F, Slack G et al 2000 Routine double treatments of superficial basal cell carcinomas using aminolaevulinic acid-based photodynamic therapy. British Journal of Dermatology 143:1270–1274

Holmes MV, Dawe RS, Ferguson J et al 2004 A randomized, double-blind, placebo-controlled study of the efficacy of tetracaine gel (Ametop) for pain relief during topical photodynamic therapy. British Journal of Dermatology 150:337–340

Horn M, Wolf P, Wulf HC et al 2003 Topical methyl aminolevulinate photodynamic therapy in patients with basal cell carcinoma prone to complications and poor cosmetic outcome with conventional treatment. British Journal of Dermatology 149:1242–1249

Karrer S, Szeimies RM, Abels C et al 1998 The use of photodynamic therapy for skin cancer. Onkologie 21:20–27

Karrer S, Szeimies RM, Hohenleutner U et al 2001 Role of lasers and photodynamic therapy in the treatment of cutaneous malignancy. American Journal of Clinical Dermatology 2:229–237

Kuijpers DIM, Smeets NWJ, Krekels GAM et al 2004 Photodynamic therapy as adjuvant treatment of extensive basal cell carcinoma treated with Mohs micrographic surgery. Dermatologic Surgery 30:794–798

Morton CA, Brown SB, Collins S et al 2002 Guidelines for topical photodynamic therapy: report of a workshop of the British Photodermatology Group. British Journal of Dermatology 146:552–567

Morton CA, MacKie RM, Whitehurst C et al 1998 Photodynamic therapy for basal cell carcinoma: effect of tumor thickness and duration of photosensitizer application on response. Archives of Dermatology 134:248–249

Morton CA 2004 Photodynamic therapy for nonmelanoma skin cancer – and more? Archives of Dermatology 140:116–120

Morton CA, Whitehurst C, McColl JH et al 2001 Photodynamic therapy for large or multiple patches of Bowen disease and basal cell carcinoma. Archives of Dermatology 137:319–324

Pagliaro J, Elliott T, Bulsara M et al 2004 Cold air analgesia in photodynamic therapy of basal cell carcinomas and Bowen's disease: an effective addition to treatment: a pilot study. Dermatologic Surgery 30:63–66

Peng Q, Warloe T, Berg K et al 1997 5-ALA based photodynamic therapy. Cancer 79:2282–2308

Rhodes LE, de Rie M, Enström Y et al 2004 Photodynamic therapy using topical methyl aminolevulinate vs surgery for nodular basal cell carcinoma. Archives of Dermatology 140:17–23

Rowe DE 1995 Comparison of treatment modalities for basal cell carcinoma. Clinical Dermatology 13:617–620

Siddiqui MAA, Perry CM, Scott LJ 2004 Topical methyl aminolevulinate. American Journal of Clinical Dermatology 5:127–137

Soler AM, Warloe T, Berner A, Giercksky KE 2001 A follow-up study of recurrence and cosmesis in completely responding superficial and nodular basal cell carcinomas treated with methyl 5-aminolaevulinate-based photodynamic therapy alone and with prior curettage. British Journal of Dermatology 145:467–471

Soler AM, Warloe T, Tausjo J et al 1999 Photodynamic therapy by topical aminolevulinic acid, dimethylsulphoxide and curettage in nodular basal cell carcinoma: a one-year follow-up study. Acta Dermato-venereologica 79:204–206

Thissen MRTM, Schroeter CA, Neumann HAM 2000 Photodynamic therapy with delta-aminolaevulinic acid for nodular basal cell carcinomas using a prior debulking technique. British Journal of Dermatology 142:338–339

Varma S, Wilson H, Kurwa HA et al 2001 Bowen's disease, solar keratoses and superficial basal cell carcinomas treated by photodynamic therapy using a large-field incoherent light source. British Journal of Dermatology 144:567–574

Wang I, Bendsoe N, Klinteberg CAF et al 2001 Photodynamic therapy vs. cryosurgery of basal cell carcinomas: results of a phase III clinical trial. British Journal of Dermatology 144:832–840

Zeitouni NC, Oseroff AR, Shieh S 2003 Photodynamic therapy for nonmelanoma skin cancers. Molecular Immunology 39:1133–1136

Treatment of Human Papilloma Virus

6

Ida Marie Stender

Introduction

The problem being treated

Based on the promising results from randomized as well nonrandomized clinical trials, this chapter will describe treatment of recalcitrant hand and foot warts with 5-aminolevulinic acid (ALA) photodynamic therapy (PDT). PDT-ALA treatment of condyloma and the human papilloma virus (HPV)-related viral condition of vulvar and vaginal intraepithelial neoplasia (VIN) will be discussed, but for these conditions, the methodology will only be generally described, since treatment modalities have not yet been standardized.

HPV in Hand and Foot Warts

Etiology

HPV is a double-stranded DNA virus of the papova virus family. It replicates within nuclei, producing hyperproliferative lesions. More than 70 genotypes of HPV have been identified. Hand and foot warts are mainly caused by HPV 1, 2, and 4, and genital warts (i.e. condylomata acuminata) by HPV 6, 11, 16, and 18.

Prevalence

The exact prevalence of warts is not known, however they are very common. About 22% of schoolchildren have warts. Up to 50–95% of renal transplant patients develop virus-associated squamous cell carcinomas (SCCs) as well as warts 5 years after transplantation.

Clinical appearance

HPV infection can present on skin as foot (i.e. plantar) and hand warts, flat warts, and genital warts. Warts can be classified by clinical appearance, location, histology and type of virus. Warts are pleomorphic and can affect skin as well as mucosa. HPV-related benign lesions may appear as papules or as nodules with a horny surface that range in size from 1 mm to several centimeters and may even become confluent to form large masses. Palmar and plantar warts are often associated with pain and may result in functional disturbances. Hand warts represent cosmetic as well as functional problems. Bothersome bleeding from finger warts may occur.

Diagnostics

Clinical judgment of an experienced dermatologist is usually sufficient for the correct diagnosis of a wart. Systematic use of standardized diagnostic criteria is of limited utility in improving diagnostic accuracy.

Histology

Hand and foot warts are characterized by hyperplasia of all layers of the epidermis. Acanthosis, papillomatosis, hyperkeratosis with parakeratosis, and thrombosed capillaries in dermal papillae are seen. Elongated ridges curve towards the center of the wart. Viral replication takes place in differentiated keratinocytes in or above the stratum granulosum. Vacuolated cells, called koilocytotic cells, are located in the mid to upper dermis.

Transmission

Warts are transmitted by direct or indirect cutaneous infection with the human papilloma virus. A defect in the stratum corneum may be a point of entry for HPV. Indirect contact with desquamated infected keratinocytes as well as autoinoculation are additional possible routes for infection.

Therapeutic challenges

Two-thirds of all hand and foot warts are never noticed by the patient and may, like many other viral infections, disappear without any therapy. Warts can however be resistant to current therapies and represent a therapeutic challenge.

Reasons for wart removal include functional, cosmetic and psychosocial concerns. The fear of developing more warts and the fear of transferring the warts to other persons are also common reasons. Although there is no fully reliable cure for virus infections such as warts, there is an intense wish from patients to be treated. The main reasons patients cite for wanting wart treatment are, respectively, the unsightly appearance, pain, and concern that the warts might spread.

Patient Selection

Patients with warts remaining after properly applied standard treatments administered by a dermatologist for more than at least 3 months may be offered PDT-ALA.

Pain during and after PDT-ALA should be considered a relative contraindication for treatment, particularly when treating children, since no effective analgesia is available.

Pregnant and nursing women should not be offered PDT-ALA because of lack of treatment experience and safety data in this subgroup.

Patients with porphyria or other photo-induced or exacerbated diseases, as well as patients allergic to the content of the ALA cream should not be offered PDT-ALA.

Expected Benefits

A series of six PDT-ALA treatments during a 9-week period has proven effective for treatment of recalcitrant warts. The treatment schedule may be refined to meet specific patient needs but extensive experience is not available with alternative protocols.

Efficacy of the treatment can be measured as the relative change in wart area after treatment as well as the treatment-related change in wart count. To evaluate whether a wart has resolved, it is convenient to assess whether the fine ridges in skin are absent at the site or not. Presence or reappearance of skin ridges indicates that the wart is no longer present. If paring reveals no capillaries, wart resolution is further confirmed. The capillaries can be easily seen by an episcope.

PDT-ALA is superior to PDT-placebo when both wart area and number of resolving warts are considered. In one double-blinded study, a total of 232 foot and hand warts in 45 patients were randomized to receive either PDT-ALA or PDT-placebo. Prior to irradiation with a broadband light source, 20% ALA cream or placebo cream was applied for 4 h, and the treatment was repeated weekly for 3 weeks. Patients were followed up 1 month later, and if warts persisted, they were retreated for a further three weekly treatments and assessed at weeks 14 and 18. Study results indicated a significant decrease in wart area in the active treatment group at weeks 14 and 18, with a median difference of 46% and 29%, respectively ($P = 0.006$, $P = 0.008$). Complete clearance of warts by week 18 was seen in 56% of patients in the active treatment group, compared with 42% in the placebo-treated group ($P < 0.05$). Both the number of resolving warts and the difference in relative wart area at weeks 14 and 18 were significant ($P < 0.05$) in favor of ALA-PDT (Tables 6.1, 6.2).

It is inconvenient for patients to come to the clinic for application of ALA-containing cream and return 3 h later for irradiation; patients, however, are easily taught how to pare the warts and how to apply the ALA cream themselves. Self-administration of ALA by the patient results in only one doctor visit, the one for irradiation, which takes about 10 min. The precise duration of irradiation depends on the number of warts to be treated as well as the number of lamps that are available. Different areas can be irradiated simultaneously, and patients are able to return to work immediately thereafter.

Compared with invasive treatment modalities, PDT-ALA has the advantage of giving excellent cosmetic results without causing damage to the surrounding skin, and permitting large areas of skin to be treated in one session.

No serious local or systemic adverse events were reported in a series of patients given six PDT-ALA treatments over 9 weeks. Scarring, other skin abnormalities, and functional disturbance were not noted. A slight, transient hyperpigmentation has been observed after removal of some warts on the dorsum of the hands and feet. Additionally, transient pain is frequently seen. Pain intensity immediately and 24 h after each intervention was assessed by a five-point scale in one study and the results are summarized in Table 6.3. A significantly higher pro-portion of the active PDT-ALA patients vs. controls experienced moderate to severe pain immediately following treatment and 24 h after light exposure.

PDT-ALA produces no plume and no bleeding, and therefore PDT-ALA reduces risk of transfer of HPV particles. The treatment is easily, routinely, and repeatedly administered on an outpatient basis without toxic side effects.

Cost /Benefit

A convenient lamp and ALA cream are needed to perform PDT-ALA. ALA cream may vary in price depending on preparation type, brand, sales channel and country of purchase. It can be prepared by the doctor or a pharmacist, or bought as a commercialized ALA product. Taking Denmark as an example in 2004, 2 g of a commercialized cream containing methyl ester ALA will cost around €200 (1 euro is

	ALA-PDT		Placebo-PDT		
Week	Persist	Vanish	Persist	Vanish	P
0	117 (100%)	0	115 (100%)	0	–
7	98 (85%)	18 (16%)	96 (84%)	19 (17%)	0.835
14	49 (50%)	49 (50%)	64 (65%)	34 (35%)	0.030
18	50 (44%)	64 (56%)	65 (58%)	47 (42%)	0.033

Number (%) of persisting and vanishing warts in ALA-PDT and placebo-PDT groups

Table 6.1 Number (%) of persisting and vanishing warts in ALA-PDT and placebo-PDT groups. Data from Stender IM, Na R, Fogh H, Gluud C, Wulff HC. Photodynamic therapy with 5-aminolaevulinic acid or placebo for recalcitrant foot and hand warts: randomised double-blind trail. Lancet 2000, 355:963–966 © 2000 Elsevier Ltd

Relative change in wart area and area of persisting warts compared with area at entry (%) at weeks 7, 14, and 18

Week No.	ALA-PDT	Placebo-PDT	Difference CI)	P
7				
Area of warts compared with area at entrance				
Median	–33	–12		0.07
Quartiles	(–74.0)	(–60.0)		
Range	(–100 to 483)	(–100 to 100)		
Area of persisting warts compared to area at entrance				
Mean change (SE)	–16.4 (6.1)	–11.2(6.1)	–5.2(19.4, 9.0)	Not significant
14				
Area of persisting warts compared with area at entrance				
Median	–98	–52		0.0006
Quartiles	(–100, –55)	(–100.0)		
Range	(–100, –56)	(–100, –25)		
Area of warts compared with area at entrance				
Mean change (SE)	–45.3(5.5)	–16.7(4.8)	–28.6(–15.9, 41.4)	0.00001
18				
Area of warts compared with area at entrance				
Median	–100	–71		0.008
Quartiles	(–100, –57)	(–100,0)		
Range	(–100 to 56)	(–100 to 60)		
Area of persisting warts compared with area at entrance				
Mean change (SE)	–38.2(6.3)	–20.1(5.3)	–18.1(–3.6, –32.6)	0.015

Table 6.2 Relative change in wart area and area of persisting warts compared with area at entry (%) at weeks 7, 14, and 18. Data from Stender IM, Na R, Fogh H, Gluud C, Wulff HC. Photodynamic therapy with 5-aminolaevulinic acid or placebo for recalcitrant foot and hand warts: randomised double-blind trail. Lancet 2000, 355:963–966 © 2000 Elsevier Ltd

Pain assessed by a five-point scale of individual warts (%) immediately and 24 h after each of six interventions					
	Pain induced by PDT-ALA				
Intervention No.	**No**	**Light**	**Moderate**	**Severe**	**Unbearable**
Pain immediately after light exposure					
1	43	28	13	15	2
2	36	11	21	26	5
3	23	21	36	15	6
4	59	15	20	4	2
5	55	13	21	7	4
6	54	20	10	12	4
Pain 24 h after light exposure					
1	67	17	15	2	–
2	56	16	18	5	5
3	50	23	21	4	2
4	76	19	6	0	–
5	77	13	5	5	5
6	68	20	2	10	–

Table 6.3 Pain assessed by a five-point scale of individual warts (%) immediately and 24 h after each of six interventions. Data from Stender IM, Na R, Fogh H, Gluud C, Wulff HC. Photodynamic therapy with 5-aminolaevulinic acid or placebo for recalcitrant foot and hand warts: randomised double-blind trail. Lancet 2000, 355:963–966 © 2000 Elsevier Ltd

approximately equal to 1 US dollar). Such a quantity may be sufficient for repeated treatments of 2–3 medium-sized warts. Commercially available non-coherent light lamps suitable for PDT range in price from €6000–19 000.

Recalcitrant warts are defined as warts that have resisted various properly applied standard treatments delivered by a dermatologist for more than 3 months. For patients with such recalcitrant warts, the spending of €200 for a 58% likelihood of cure within a few weeks is an attractive trade-off. Patients with recalcitrant warts are often frustrated by multiple treatment visits over months to years, and have often failed numerous prior conventional and unconventional treatments.

The cost–benefit analysis pertaining to PDT for new and not recalcitrant warts is less obvious. The trade-offs depend on the patient and the circumstances. If the patient is not particularly bothered and the warts are likely to disappear spontaneously or within few doctor visits, the additional expenditures for PDT-ALA may not be justified.

In most countries, public health systems or various health insurance schemes are setting guidelines for which therapies can be used and what trade-offs can be made between patient satisfaction and spending. Most such schemes, however, do not take into account the total cost of wart treatment. In addition

to direct medical costs, indirect but significant costs such as lost work time, travel time to and from clinics for patients and accompanying relatives, and the spreading of the virus to others may not be considered by policymakers. In the narrow traditional cost–benefit perspective, the additional cost of ALA is typically only compared to the likely cost of additional patient- and physician-administered therapies (salicylic acid-containing ointments, cryotherapy, curettage, cantharidine etc.) that may be required. Since the exact number of required visits for wart treatment may be unknown, such trade-off analyses tend to be biased towards whichever treatment modality is cheapest per treatment. Since a traditional therapy often employs relatively inexpensive medications, PDT is still often excluded by health insurance schemes. As PDT is an emerging therapy, its availability is expected to increase over time as its cumulative efficacy becomes apparent and the unit cost of treatment is reduced over time by improved technology and volume-related savings.

For the dermatologist, the curing of a patient in fewer visits entails a superior use of resources. However, if the dermatologist is not paid for offering PDT either by the patient or by the health system, there is no incentive to invest in PDT lamps(s), train personnel or acquire and administer the more expensive ALA medication. Needless to say, the treatment modalities for recalcitrant warts most favored by clinic administrators are those that maximize fee generation while requiring little investment.

Wart removal has traditionally not been among the most prestigious dermatological skills, but for the patients affected with this troublesome, often intractable problem, an expeditious cure is highly valued.

Condyloma and Intraepithelial Neoplasia

Condyloma acuminata is a very common sexually transmitted disease for which no treatment is completely satisfactory. HPV infection with certain oncogenic viral types can lead to the development of intraepithelial neoplasia (IN) of the cervix, vagina, vulva, and anus.

Diagnosis of condyloma is made by vulvoscopy following 2% acetic acid application, and diagnosis of IN is made by biopsy. The most common site for condyloma are the perineal skin, periclitorial area and labia minora, where multifocal or confluent areas vary in size, color and appearance. The affected cutaneous surface is often irregular, warty and ulcerated. Of all IN lesions, 20% are asymptomatic; however, the most common presenting symptom is pruritus. Diagnosis is based upon full-thickness biopsy.

Conventional treatment for condyloma involves various topical medications, cryotherapy and laser, whereas the treatment of VIN often may involve local surgical excision with wide margins and laser ablation.

PDT-ALA is a treatment for condylomata acuminata, with an overall cure rate of 72.9% (ALA 20% cream, irradiation with optical system made at Forth-IESL, 400–800 nm, 70–100 J/cm^2, 70 mW/cm^{-2}). In one protocol, ALA gel (10%) was applied to vulvar and vaginal lesions followed by occlusion with a dressing for a mean interval of 154 min and ultimate illumination with a 635 nm dye laser. Evaluation after 2 months revealed clearance of lesions in 66–73% of the condyloma patients and 37–57% of patients with IN. Young age and multifocal disease are associated with a high recurrence rate. PDT-ALA seems to have efficacy similar to that of conventional treatments, while healing time is shorter and preservation of normal morphology excellent. The low recurrence rate following PDT may be due to effective treatment of small, subclinical microscopic foci.

In sum, ALA-PDT is a noninvasive, easy to perform, minimally tissue destructive, well-tolerated modality with excellent cosmetic results and abbreviated healing time compared to laser treatment.

Mechanism Behind Antiviral Effect of PDT

PDT acts in HPV infection mainly by the destruction of infected keratinocytes and inactivation of viral particles of nonenveloped viruses. Photosensitizer molecules may bind to the viral surface glycoproteins, resulting in an inhibition of the early phases of viral infection. Significantly, the penetration depth of ALA and light may be a limiting factor for treatment of thick lesions such as warts. The callus of warts should therefore be removed before ALA cream application. Virus-containing keratinocytes, which are located in the upper epidermis within or above stratum granulosum, are similar in situation to superficial basal cell carcinomas (BCCs) that are reportedly successfully treated with PDT. Thus, although warts are thick epidermal lesions, after paring, the infected keratinocytes may be reached by light and ALA.

Overview of Treatment Strategy for Hand and Foot Warts (Fig. 6.1)

Treatment approach – major determinants

Photodynamic therapy is documented to be effective for treatment of common warts. Preliminary reports also indicate successful treatment of other similar lesions, including flat warts, mosaic warts, warts in immunosuppressed patients, and genital warts.

The active photosensitizer ALA may be prepared in different ways. A 20% aminolevulinic acid-containing cream prepared in the local hospital pharmacy was used in one double-blinded treatment study of warts. However, due to its lipophilic nature, methylesteraminolevulinic acid (PDT-MAL) has an increased diffusion across cell membranes, which may lead to a deeper penetration and therefore a more effective treatment of deeper lesions. Furthermore, studies have shown that pain induced by PDT-MAL is less than that associated with PDT-ALA. MAL is marketed under the Metvix label in Europe (since 2000 in Denmark).

The penetration of light into wart tissue is limited to a few millimeters and increases with increasing

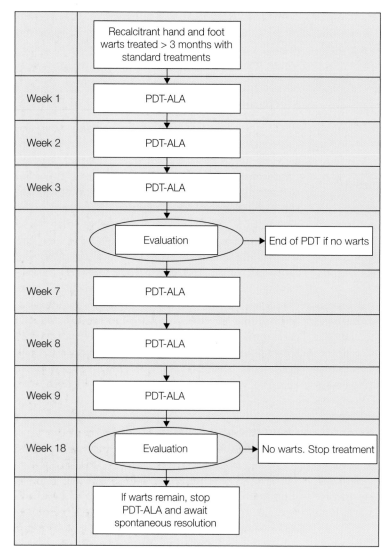

	Recalcitrant hand and foot warts treated > 3 months with standard treatments
Week 1	PDT-ALA
Week 2	PDT-ALA
Week 3	PDT-ALA
	Evaluation → End of PDT if no warts
Week 7	PDT-ALA
Week 8	PDT-ALA
Week 9	PDT-ALA
Week 18	Evaluation → No warts. Stop treatment
	If warts remain, stop PDT-ALA and await spontaneous resolution

Fig. 6.1 PDT flowchart: An overview of Treatment Strategy for Hand and Foot Warts

wavelength. An appropriate light source for PDT-ALA emits light in a wavelength range including the absorption peaks of PpIX. Lasers as well as nonlaser light sources can be used.

Light sources used for PDT vary from slide projectors to xenon, halogen, and tungsten lamps, as well as advanced lasers. The optimal wavelength of light, whether it is applied as a low dose for a relatively long exposure time or as a high dose for short exposure time, is not still well defined. Total energy doses for PDT light sources have also not been standardized and may vary from 60–250 J/cm² for laser lights and for 30–540 J/cm² for nonlasers. In one study, warts were exposed to a fluence of 50 mW/cm² for 23 min, which corresponded to a total dose of 70 J/cm².

For PDT-ALA treatment of HPV-induced warts a commonly used and effective light source is the commercially available Waldmann PDT 1200 lamp (Waldmann-Medizin-technik, Villingen-Schwenningen, Germany) that emits in the range 590–700 nm, including the PpIX absorption peaks at 630 nm and 690 nm. Another useful light device is the Photocure lamp (Photocure of Norway). The Photocure lamp has an elegant design, and is portable and easy to use with a built-in cooling fan. A convenient version of the lamp is mounted on the wall or ceiling and a small table model exists as well. Having several of these

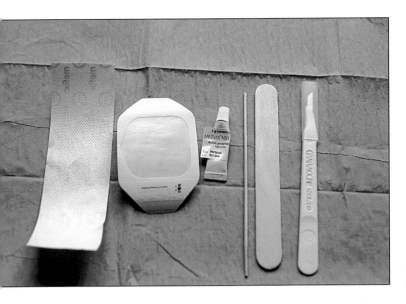

Fig. 6.2 Bandage, foil, ALA cream, application tools and scalpel

lamps in the clinic enables the treatment of several warts simultaneously.

Treatment Techniques for Hand and Foot Warts

Patients

Not all wart patients need to be treated. Indications for treatment are pain, interference with functioning or cosmetic embarrassment. Patients with recalcitrant hand and foot warts that had been offered various unsuccessful treatments should be offered PDT-ALA.

Equipment

- 20% ALA (Sigma Co, St Louis, MO, USA) prepared in a cream base, Metvix, or similar formulation
- Lamp (e.g. Waldmann, Photocure, or tungsten and other convenient lamps)
- Scalpel
- Bandages
- Spray bottle for water-cooling.

Treatment algorithm

During the 18-week period for PDT-ALA treatment, patients are expected to pare their warts with a scalpel and apply keratolytics twice a week.

No local anesthesia is needed before treatment of warts with PDT-ALA.

Paring of warts and application of ALA cream can be performed by patient or nurse. Few concurrent treatments are required while patients are undergoing PDT treatment (Fig. 6.2):

1. The warts are pared with a scalpel to remove the horny layer (while avoiding bleeding) prior to ALA cream application (Fig. 6.3). In case of bleeding, treatment should be deferred until bleeding has stopped.
2. Apply a visible layer of ALA-containing cream on the warts and to a 0.5–1 cm margin beyond the warts (Figs 6.4, 6.5).
3. Cover the warts with a foil or occlusive dressing (e.g. Tegaderm R, 3M) (Fig. 6.6).
4. Cover the dressing with extra fixation when Mefix is used. Apply the Mefix bandage to the lateral side of the feet to avoid loosening when the patient walks (Fig. 6.7).

Patients can apply the cream in the morning and come to the clinic for irradiation 3–4 h later during their lunch break. Some patients prefer to apply the cream at 5:00 a.m. and come for irradiation on their way to work.

Irradiation is performed 3–4 h later by a nurse as follows:

1. Remove the bandages and ointment (Fig. 6.8).

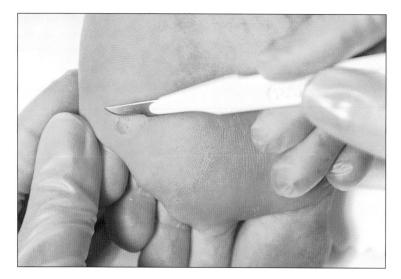

Fig. 6.3 Paring of wart with scalpel

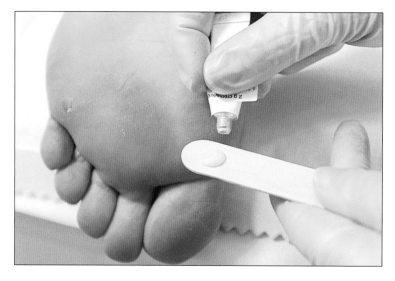

Fig. 6.4 Use a spatula for reasons of hygiene

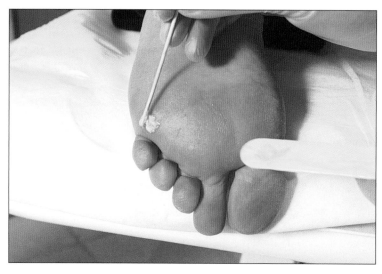

Fig. 6.5 Apply a visible layer of cream to the lesion

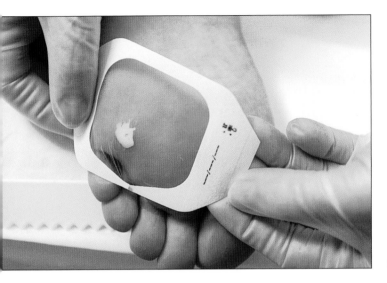

Fig. 6.6 Wart being covered by foil

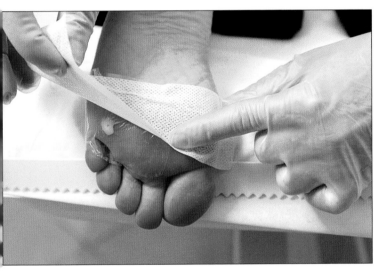

Fig. 6.7 Extra fixation bandage

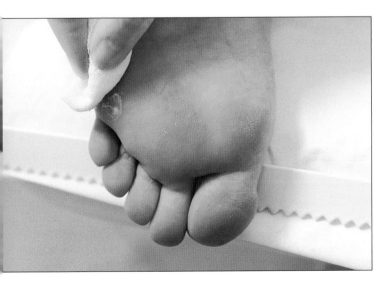

Fig. 6.8 Removal of bandage

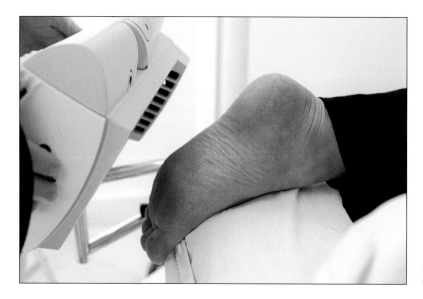

Fig. 6.9 Place lamp in right position depending on lamp

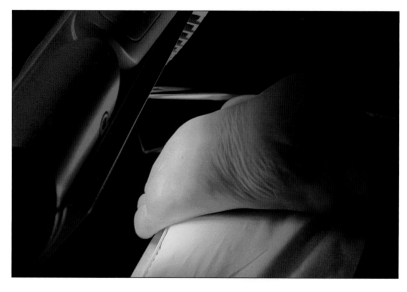

Fig. 6.10 Irradiation for 7 min (depending on lamp). (Photocure lamp: 7 min, 570–670 nm, 75 J/cm²)

2. Patient and nurse should use protecting glasses during the irradiation period since the red light can irritate the eyes.

3. Place the lamp in the correct position and start illumination. Using the Photocure Cure light, appropriate parameters are a distance of 8–11 cm from the wart (Fig. 6.9) with irradiation (570–670 nm, 75 J/cm²) for 7 min (Fig. 6.10). Using the PDT Waldmann 1200, the parameters are 590–700 nm, 50 mW/cm² for 23 min (70 J/cm²). Make the patient as comfortable as possible given the location of the warts (Fig. 6.11). In case of pain, apply water with a spray bottle (Fig. 6.12). If pain relief is not sufficient,

increase the distance from the light to the irradiated area or take breaks during the irradiation procedure.

4. Turn the light off when the proper dose has been given.

5. Treated lesions should be protected against direct sun and direct light during the following 48 h.

Special post-treatment care, except avoiding light exposure, is not necessary. As per previous studies, the earlier described PDT procedure should be repeated three times with 1-week intervals between treatment; then, 1 month of observation should, in case of persisting warts, be followed by three more

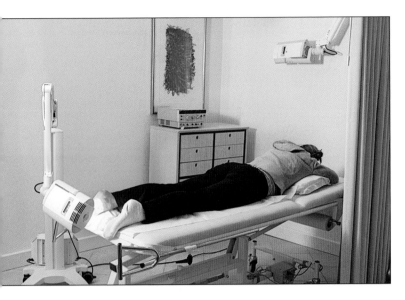

Fig. 6.11 Position the patient comfortably for the irradiation period

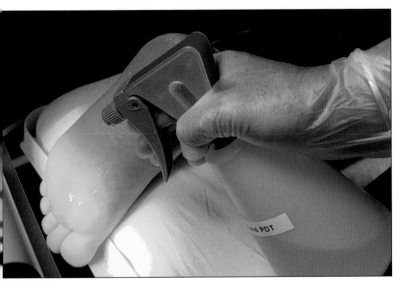

Fig. 6.12 Spray water to soothe pain

PDT treatments. After the last treatment, patients should continue to pare their warts twice a week followed by local application of a keratolytic. The final evaluation of the effect should take place 2 months after the last treatment.

Troubleshooting

Final evaluation of the effect too soon after the last PDT treatment may lead to disappointing results. Do not evaluate response before 2 months after the last PDT treatment.

Multiple PDT treatments are needed. One treatment is not effective.

Preparation of the warts before treatment as well as home treatment by the patient is necessary.

Side effects, complications, and alternative approaches

Pain during PDT shows wide inter-patient variance.

Pain is one of the major side effects of PDT-ALA. Some patients do benefit from systemic analgesia before and after PDT treatment. If burning and stinging occurs during and after PDT treatment, application of cold water may help to relieve the pain. Usually pain resolves within 48 h after irradiation of the warts. Pain post-treatment can be treated with anti-inflammatory agents and with cooling down of the treated lesion with ice.

During irradiation the pain may be unacceptable in about 10% of the lesions treated. If this occurs, light intensity may be reduced by increasing the distance from the lamp to the warts. In case this maneuver is not sufficient, briefer light therapy may be delivered.

Severe complications after PDT treatment are extremely rare. Healing is almost invariably without scar formation.

Only patients who have tried various conventional and nonconventional wart treatments are treated with ALA-PDT. Resistance of warts to treatment may be mitigated by paring, but additional co-treatments should be avoided to prevent excessive irritation.

It is a valid management option to leave warts untreated.

Further Reading

El-Said A-H, Martin-Hirsch P, Duggan-Keen M et al 2001 Immunological and viral factors associated with the response of vulval intraepithelial neoplasia to photodynamic therapy. Cancer Research 61:192–196

Fabbrocini G, Di Constanzo MP, Riccardo AM et al 2001 Photodynamic therapy with topical δ-aminolaevulinic acid for the treatment of plantar warts. Journal of Photochemistry and Photobiology B: Biology 61:30–34

Fehr MK, Hornung R, Degen A et al 2002 Photodynamic therapy of vulvar and vaginal condyloma and intrapithelial neoplasia using topically applied 5-aminolevulinic acid. Lasers in Surgery and Medicine 30:273–279

Ibbotson SH 2002 Topical 5-aminolaevulinic acid photodynamic therapy for the treatment of skin conditions other than non-melanoma skin cancer. British Journal of Dermatology 146:178–188

Stefanaki IM, Georgiou S, Themelis GC et al 2003 In vivo fluorescence kinetics and photodynamic therapy in condylomata acuminata. British Journal of Dermatology 149:972–976

Stender IM, Na R, Fogh H et al 2000 Photodynamic therapy with 5-aminolaevulinic acid or placebo for recalcitrant foot and hand warts: randomised double-blind trial. The Lancet 355:963–966

7

Other Dermatologic Indications for ALA-PDT

Erin M. Welch, Kristen Kelly

Introduction

Topical 5-aminolevulinic acid (ALA) photodynamic therapy (PDT) is a relatively simple technique, has a low risk of serious side effects and results in a good cosmetic outcome. As such, its efficacy has been evaluated for a wide range of dermatologic disorders.

The mechanism of tissue injury following topical application of ALA has been discussed in depth in earlier chapters. Briefly, topically applied ALA is capable of penetrating through the stratum corneum (with penetration significantly enhanced in abnormal keratin) and is accumulated in certain cell populations, including some lymphocyte groups. Nonfluorescent, nonphotodynamically active ALA is then transformed into highly fluorescent and photodynamically active protoporphyrin IX (PpIX) via

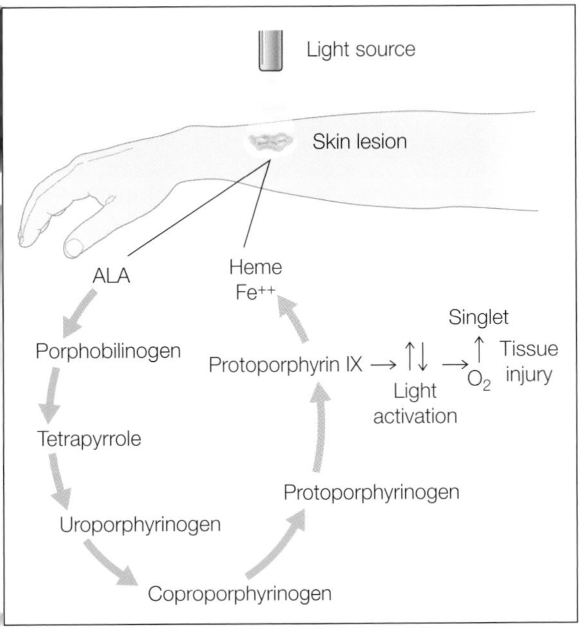

Fig. 7.1 Schematic diagram of the mechanism of photodynamic therapy using topically applied aminolevulinic acid

the heme cycle (Fig. 7.1). PpIX can be activated by light and excited to a higher energy level. The energy is then transferred to tissue oxygen resulting in generation of cytotoxic singlet oxygen species, which causes tissue damage. In this manner, a photochemical reaction creates injury as opposed to the heat-induced effects typically observed during many light–tissue interactions.

Cutaneous T-cell lymphomas and psoriasis have been the focus of several studies, while a few case reports have evaluated the utility of ALA-PDT for lichen sclerosus, lichen planus, scleroderma and vascular tumors. These applications of ALA-PDT are less widely utilized than those discussed in earlier chapters and treatment protocols are not clearly established. However, patients with these conditions who have resistant localized disease, lesions in difficult anatomic locations or are unable to tolerate alternative treatments because of adverse effects, may benefit from ALA-PDT.

Cutaneous T-cell Lymphoma

The problem being treated

Cutaneous T-cell lymphoma is a malignant neoplasm of T-lymphocytes, specifically T-helper cells. It is a chronic disease with wide variability in rate of progression and aggressiveness. Lesions of cutaneous T-cell lymphoma may be differentiated by clinical appearance into stages, including patch, plaque, tumor or erythroderma. Early lesions may resemble a variety of dermatoses and can be described as eczematous, erythematous or psoriasiform. Accurate diagnosis requires clinical and histologic correlation. Systemic involvement portends a significantly worse prognosis and requires aggressive systemic treatment. However, many patients have localized disease that may remain as such for years, during

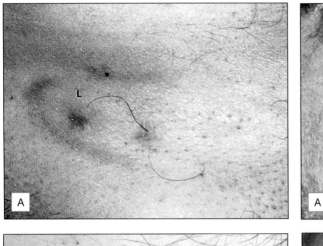

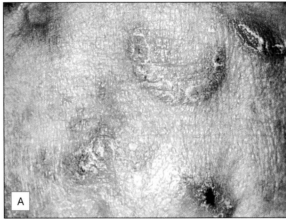

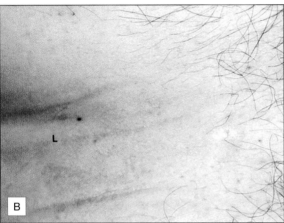

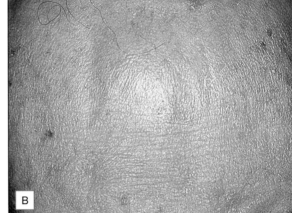

Fig. 7.2 Cutaneous T-cell lymphoma lesion of the abdomen (**A**) before treatment and (**B**) 6 months after topical ALA-PDT, 170 J/cm². (Photographs courtesy of Arie Orenstein, Genady Kostenich, and Dermatologic Surgery)

Fig. 7.3 Nodular cutaneous T-cell lymphoma on the forehead (**A**) before treatment and (**B**) 6 months after topical ALA-PDT, 340–380 J/cm². (Photographs courtesy of Arie Orenstein, Genady Kostenich, and Dermatologic Surgery)

which only limited cutaneous therapy and careful monitoring are required.

Topical ALA-PDT has been used for treatment of localized cutaneous T-cell lymphoma (Figs 7.2, 7.3). The rationale for this treatment approach was provided by early evaluations by Boehncke et al, which demonstrated selective photosensitizer uptake into lesions of mycosis fungoides during topical PDT with subsequent inhibition of malignant transformed T cells. Other studies, for example by Orenstein et al, indicated that malignant blood cells have an increased ability to convert ALA into PP (protoporphyrin) as compared to normal blood cells.

Patient selection

Patients with T-cell lymphoma limited to the skin are candidates for ALA-PDT. Many treatment options are available for cutaneous T-cell lymphoma including topical corticosteroids, topical nitrogen mustard, retinoids, psoralen in combination with UV irradiation (PUVA), radiation therapy, excision and carbon dioxide laser surgery. Each of these therapies has limitations related to adverse effects or efficacy, and as such, alternatives are often sought. Topical ALA-PDT offers an additional treatment strategy that may be especially useful in patients with difficult-to-treat lesions because of localized resistance, problematic location or other health considerations.

Expected benefits

Complete clinical remission of localized cutaneous T-cell lymphoma has been achieved with ALA-PDT, although this is not the case for all lesions (Table 7.1).

Parameters for treatment of cutaneous T-cell lymphoma with topical ALA-PDT

Reference	No. of sites	Application time	Wavelength (nm)	Intensity (mW/cm²)	Fluence (J/cm²)	No. of Rx	Lesion type	Response[a]	Recurrence
Coors 2004	7	6 h	Visible light	60–160	72–144	1–7	5 plaque 2 tumor	CCR all lesions	None at 14–18 months
Edstrom 2001	12	5–18 h	600–730	35–320	80–180	2–11	10 plaque 2 tumor	7/10 plaque: CCR 2/10 plaque: Regression 1/10 plaque: No response 2/2 tumor: No response	None in lesions with CCR after 4–19 months
Leman 2002	2	6–24 h	630	48	100	4	Plaque	CCR all lesions	None at 12 months
Markham 2001	1	4 h	580–740	20	20	5	Tumor	CCR	None at 1 year
Orenstein 2000	6	16 h	580–720	140	170 patch 380 tumor	1	1 patch 5 tumor	CCR all lesions	None at 24 months
Oseroff 1996	80	overnight	630	30–150	10–200	1	Not specified	Varied with fluence and intensity	Not reported
Wang 1999	3	4–6 h	635	<110	60	3	Periocular	CCR all lesions	None at 33 months

[a]CCR = complete clinical response

Table 7.1 Parameters for treatment of cutaneous T-cell lymphoma with topical ALA-PDT

Prolonged remission may occur and lack of recurrence has been reported during follow up for periods as long as 2–3 years. However, it is also important to note that on occasion, clinical resolution may be observed, but biopsy may reveal persistent malignant lymphocytic infiltration. This may be most common when lesions appear to clear after one treatment. Close and frequent post-treatment monitoring is required.

Treatment techniques

As documented in Table 7.1, a range of treatment strategies has been utilized for topical ALA-PDT of cutaneous T-cell lymphoma. The best protocol has not yet been established. Several factors affect treatment outcome, including photosensitizer concentration and application time, light dose, light intensity, lesion stage or thickness and anatomic location.

20% ALA has commonly been utilized in successful clinical trials. A variety of application times have been investigated, but in many patients, a period of 4–6 h appears to be adequate, especially when the area is occluded (generally with a light-shielding dressing).

A study by Oseroff et al evaluated the effect of light dose and intensity on clinical effectiveness. They found that clinical efficacy increased with fluence (starting at $10 \, J/cm^2$), reaching a plateau at $75–100 \, J/cm^2$. Intensity also affected treatment response. In general, an intensity of $150 \, mW/cm^2$ caused the least epidermal damage and was more effective than lower fluence rates.

A study by Edstrom et al noted the effects of fluence, intensity and lesional area on treatment tolerance. They started with a fluence of $180 \, J/cm^2$ but later in their study treatment fluence was halved, secondary to pain. They also found that patients were not able to tolerate very high intensities ($200–320 \, mW/cm^2$), and in many patients, an intensity of $35–125 \, mW/cm^2$ achieved a good clinical outcome. In their conclusions, they recommended avoidance of very high intensities to diminish patient discomfort and improve compliance with further treatments. Finally, they noted that treatment of larger areas resulted in greater pain.

Fractionation may improve results, especially in thick lesions. Orenstein et al used a 30-minute irradiation session ($580–720 \, nm$, $140 \, mW/cm^2$, $252 \, J/cm^2$) followed by a 1-hour dark period and then a second 10–15 min of irradiation (total cumulative dose $340–380 \, J/cm^2$) for 1–4 mm-deep tumor stage lesions. Leman et al theorized that fractionation might allow oxygen replenishment and improve the efficiency of the photodynamic process.

Orenstein et al also found that on-line in vivo fluorescence monitoring (Figs 7.4, 7.5) may be a useful tool for determining optimal light dosing. For fluorescence detection, they used blue light (400–450 nm, $20 \, mW/cm^2$) delivered by an optical fiber. A CCIR camera was used for imaging and a CCD-based fiberoptic spectrometer (spectral range 570–720 nm, spectral resolution 10 nm) was used for assessment of fluorescence signal intensity. Fluorescence imaging and spectroscopy were performed pre-treatment, during treatment and then 1 h after treatment. If PP fluorescence recurred (frequently seen in thicker lesions), re-treatment was considered until fluorescence was significantly diminished or eliminated.

A study by Wang et al evaluated the use of ALA-PDT for lesions in difficult-to-treat anatomic areas, specifically those in the periocular region. Such lesions may be ideal opportunities for the use of ALA-PDT, although special procedures and precautions may be required. One patient had three lesions on the medial canthus and lower eyelids bilaterally and failed nine cycles of chemotherapy. Eyedrops were used to anesthetize the eye, followed by cleansing and removal of lesional debris with

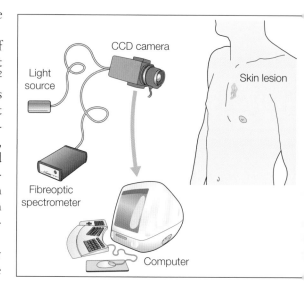

Fig. 7.4 Schematic diagram of fluorescence monitoring during ALA-PDT treatment

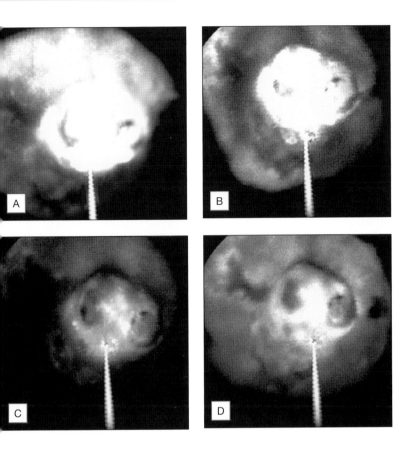

Fig. 7.5 Typical fluorescence images of a nodular cutaneous T-cell lymphoma lesion. (**A**) 16 h after topical ALA application. (**B**) After 10 min of light exposure. (**C**) After 30 min of light exposure. (**D**) Recovery after 1 h of photoprotection. (Photographs courtesy of Arie Orenstein, Genady Kostenich, and Dermatologic Surgery)

normal saline. The eye to be treated was covered with a specially designed lead shield placed intra-orbitally. The lesion surface was then gently scraped with a scalpel to improve ALA penetration. Curetting of the lesion was not performed as this can increase the pain of the procedure and may result in scarring. ALA powder (Porphyrin Products, Logan, UT, USA) was dissolved in neutral eye ointment (Emulgon) to achieve a concentration of 20% ALA. The ointment was applied to the lesion and a 5 mm peripheral margin and covered with a thin adhesive plastic pad (Tegaderm, 3M, UK). A complete clinical response (CCR) and excellent cosmetic result with no scarring was achieved after three treatments. Follow-up for 33 months revealed no recurrence.

A study by Coors et al demonstrated the utility of topical ALA-PDT for treatment of cutaneous T-cell lymphoma lesions resistant to other therapies. Seven previously resistant lesions were treated with 20% 5-ALA under occlusion for 6 h followed by visible light irradiation. A complete remission was achieved in all lesions.

Side effects and complications

Moderate to severe discomfort during treatment is common. Leman et al used intralesional anesthetics or a water spray during treatment to improve tolerability while Coors and von den Driesch used liquid nitrogen sprayed repeatedly in the air about 10 cm above the treated lesion. Pagliaro et al reported using cold-air analgesia to improve comfort during PDT. The post-treatment period generally includes erythema, edema and epidermal sloughing. Erosion and ulceration may occur. Lesions generally heal with a good cosmetic outcome, although pigmentary change and scarring can result. Characteristic of PDT for any indication, post-treatment photosensitivity occurs, and light protection practices are important for approximately 48 h following therapy.

Summary

Further work is required to optimize ALA-PDT treatment parameters for cutaneous T-cell lymphoma. However, this appears to be a viable treatment option, with success reported in a significant number of patients. Patients with difficult-to-treat lesions because of localized resistance, location or other health considerations, may be optimal candidates. Careful monitoring for systemic disease or local recurrence is important for all patients with cutaneous T-cell lymphoma and must be included in any treatment strategy.

Psoriasis

The problem being treated

Psoriasis is a polygenic inflammatory disorder affecting approximately 2% of the world's population. Psoriasis is clinically characterized by erythematous plaques with silvery white scales, favoring the extensor surfaces, elbows, knees, scalp, and trunk. Histologically, psoriasis lesions demonstrate hyperkeratosis, parakeratosis, acanthosis, dilated blood vessels in the papillary dermis, and an inflammatory infiltrate composed mostly of lymphocytes.

Topical and orally administered ALA have been shown by Stringer et al and Bissonette et al to be taken up selectively into psoriasis plaques and converted to PP. Interestingly, fluorescence emission was seen in psoriatic plaques up to 1 week after topical ALA application. Fluorescence was also noted at distant psoriatic plaques to which no ALA had been applied, although serum porphyrins were not detected.

Bissonnette et al recently demonstrated apoptosis in T lymphocytes of some psoriatic plaques after oral administration of ALA. This is an important observation as T lymphocytes appear to be a central factor in the pathogenesis of psoriasis and thus, successful treatment will likely require manipulation of this cell population.

Patient selection

Psoriasis can be successfully treated with many medications, including topical vitamin D derivatives, topical steroids, oral and topical retinoids, methotrexate, immunosuppressive agents such as cyclosporine, and the relatively new class of biologics. Despite these many options, many patients do not achieve complete, long-term control of their psoriasis, or experience unacceptable adverse effects. As such, alternative treatment options are often sought.

PUVA and ultraviolet B (UVB) light are frequently utilized therapies with well-proven efficacy. However, these treatments impose an increased risk of skin malignancy and generally the majority of the body is exposed. PDT may offer a light-based treatment alternative for patients with resistant psoriasis (Fig. 7.6). Optimal candidates are those patients with localized psoriatic plaques that have been resistant to topical medications and who do not require or want systemic therapies with their associated potential for adverse effects.

Expected benefits

In some patients, rapid control of resistant plaques can be achieved. Prolonged remission may be possible but, as discussed later, optimization of treatment strategies needs to occur to achieve this on a consistent basis.

Treatment techniques

Like cutaneous T-cell lymphoma, a range of treatment strategies has been utilized for ALA-PDT treatment of psoriasis (Table 7.2) and the best protocol is not yet established. Several factors affect treatment outcome and have been studied, including ALA concentration and application time, lesion thickness and number of treatments. Light wavelength, intensity and dose are also likely to be important. Oral administration of ALA for PDT has been attempted and will be discussed.

A study by Weinstein et al looked at topical ALA-PDT for psoriasis utilizing differing ALA concentrations (2%, 10% and 20%) in combination with UVA ($15\,mW/cm^2$, $2.5–3\,J/cm^2$). The best results were noted with 10% and 20% ALA, which were associated with greater than 50% improvement after four weekly treatments.

A study by Fritsch et al evaluated varying topical ALA application times and demonstrated the highest porphyrin accumulation in psoriatic lesions after 6 h, thus concluding this duration of exposure may be optimal. Fritsch and others have found in psoriatic plaques variable PpIX accumulation, which may diminish treatment efficacy. Hyperkeratosis of psoriatic lesions may be one factor limiting ALA penetration and as such, anti-keratolytic measures prior to ALA application may be beneficial. Application of keratolytics needs to be done cautiously, as significant irritation of the area will increase treatment pain and may increase the risk of other adverse effects.

A study by Collins et al demonstrated the potential for rapid clearing of psoriasis plaques. They

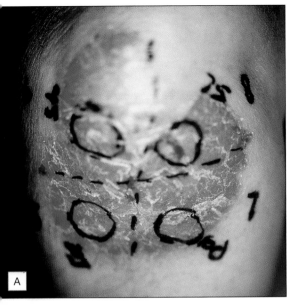

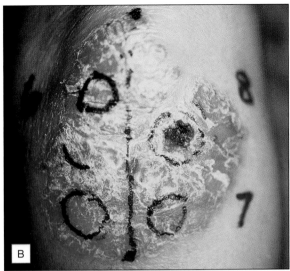

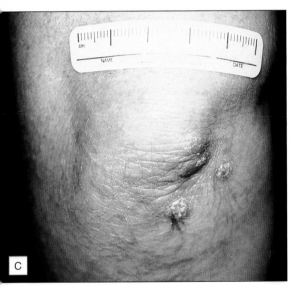

Fig. 7.6 Psoriasis plaque (**A**) before, (**B**) 2 weeks post-treatment, (**C**) 3 months post-PDT treatment. (Photographs courtesy of J.S. Nelson)

treated 36 trunk and extremity sites with 20% topical ALA applied for 4 h and irradiated with 400–650 nm light from a modified slide projector, at 10–40 mW/cm², for a total fluence of 2–16 J/cm². At evaluation 11–17 d after treatment, seven of the 22 test subjects showed improvement, with 10 of the 36 treated lesions completely clearing and four reducing up to 50% after only one treatment. However, lesions began to recur within 2 weeks.

Regimens with multiple planned treatments may achieve greater success. This was demonstrated by Robinson et al, who evaluated 19 sites after topical 20% ALA applied for 4 h followed by broad-band visible radiation with a modified slide projector (15 mW/cm², 2–8 J/cm²). Up to 12 treatments were performed one to three times a week. Eight of the 10 patients improved, with four of the 19 sites resolving completely.

It has been proposed that oral ALA-PDT may offer advantages over topical ALA-PDT in treatment of psoriasis. Bissonnette et al exposed patients to a blue fluorescent lamp at 9–11 mW/cm² using fluences up to 20 J/cm² after a period of 1–6 h following ingestion of 5, 10, or 15 mg of ALA. PpIX fluorescence increased rapidly and significantly in psoriatic plaques, reaching a maximum at 2–3 h.

Parameters for treatment of psoriasis with ALA-PDT								
Reference	No. of sites	ALA Administration	Wavelength (nm)	Intensity (mW/cm^2)	Fluence (J/cm^2)	No. of Rx	Response	Recurrence
Bissonnette 2002	180	1,3,6 h Oral	417	9–11	1–20	1	0–42%	Not reported
Boehnke 1994	3	5 Topical	600–700	70	25	3+	Partial clearance	Not reported
Robinson 1999	19	4 h Topical	Broadband visible	15	2–8	7–12	4 lesions clear, 10 improved, 5 no change	Not reported
Collins 1997	36	4 h Topical	400–650	10–40	2–16	1	10 lesions clear 4 30–50% reduction 22 no change	5–14 d later
Weinstein 1994	84	3 h Topical	Ultraviolet A	15	2.5–3	1–4	Variable improvement	Not reported

Table 7.2 Parameters for treatment of psoriasis with ALA-PDT

Maximal improvement (42% diminution in psoriasis severity score at 28 d as compared to baseline) was seen in patients who received 10 or 15 mg of ALA followed after 3 h by 10 J/cm^2 of blue light.

Side effects and complications

Patients undergoing topical ALA-PDT for psoriasis frequently experience pain, burning, and itching during and up to 72 h post-treatment. Severity of symptoms ranges from mild to severe. Post-treatment effects may also include erythema, mild edema, and occasionally erosions, especially at higher light doses. Post-inflammatory hyperpigmentation has been shown to occur often with plaque resolution, although scarring is generally not reported.

Use of oral ALA-PDT may overcome some of these issues. Bissonnette reported that treatment was well tolerated with only one patient (who received 15 mg) reporting a mild burning sensation during light exposure. Asymptomatic erythema and edema of 3 days duration were the only symptoms observed post-treatment. While administration of oral ALA has been associated with nausea, vomiting and hypotension, the 5, 10 or 15 mg doses used by Bissonnette et al resulted in only one of 12 patients reporting mild nausea.

Of course, photosensitivity after both topical and oral ALA administration and the need for light protection practices must be discussed with patients prior to treatment.

Summary

Pain and unpredictable response are the major limitations of topical ALA-PDT treatment of psoriasis at this time. Oral ALA-PDT appears to be well tolerated and offers the advantage of making treatment of larger body surface areas more practical. Photosensitivity following treatment is also an issue but may be tolerated if optimization of treatment strategy results in consistent and rapid improvement of resistant plaques. Further research is required to better evaluate the treatment potential of ALA-PDT for psoriasis.

Other Potential Indications for ALA-PDT

Lichen sclerosus et atrophicus

Lichen sclerosus et atrophicus is a chronic skin disease characterized by atrophic areas, flat, white, angular papules (often with a surrounding erythematous or violaceous halo) and follicular plugging. The anogenital area is a common location of involvement and severe itching is a frequent complaint. One study evaluated the use of ALA-PDT in an attempt to help patients with this often treatment-resistant disorder. A study by Hillemanns et al used 20% ALA applied 4–6 h, followed by irradiation with a 635 nm argon ion-pumped dye laser (40–70 mW/cm^2, 80 J/cm^2) for up to three cycles of treatment over 1–3 weeks in 12 patients. Treatment was tolerated, although vulvar erythema occurred in most patients and burning pain during therapy required opioid pain control in three patients. All experienced relief of pruritic symptoms lasting a mean of 6.1 months after therapy. Visual improvement of the lesional area was seen in only two of the patients.

Lichen planus

Lichen planus is an inflammatory, pruritic disease of the skin characterized by small, flat, purple, polygonal papules. Kirby et al was successfully treated lichen planus in one patient with a penile lesion. Over 6 weeks, he was given two cycles of 20% ALA applied for 4 h, then irradiated by a light source of 607–657 nm (55 mW/cm^2, 50 J/cm^2), resulting in clearance lasting 6 months. Improvement was thought to be secondary to an apoptotic effect of ALA-PDT on inflammatory T cells.

Scleroderma

Localized scleroderma is characterized by sclerotic changes and excess collagen formation in the skin. Five patients with 23 lesions unresponsive to steroids, systemic penicillamine, and other light therapies were treated in a study by Karrer et al with 3% ALA applied for 6 h followed by exposure to an incoherent light source (PDT 1200, Waldmann, Germany, 40 mW/cm^2, 10 J/cm^2) weekly or biweekly for 25–43 sessions. Minor stinging sensations occurred during treatment and mild hyperpigmentation was noted post-treatment. All patients showed improvement clinically as well as in quantitative measurements of skin hardness by a durometer, with changes persisting 2 years after therapy. Four of five patients had untreated control lesions elsewhere on their bodies that did not improve.

The mechanism of this interesting effect on scleroderma is uncertain. Studies of ALA and red light exposure on human dermal fibroblasts demonstrated increased production of matrix metalloproteinase-1 (MMP) and MMP-3 collagenase mRNA and reduced collagen I mRNA. ALA-PDT may also have an apoptotic effect on inflammatory cells.

Vascular lesions

PDT is an interesting therapeutic option for select vascular lesions. Port wine stains (PWSs) are congenital, vascular malformations of the skin found in approximately 0.3% of children. PWSs may be located anywhere on the body but are commonly found on the face and neck, where they may have serious psychological consequences. Others often perceive patients as 'marked', which may adversely affect personality development. Over time, these lesions may hypertrophy and patients may experience local bleeding. For these reasons, patients or their families often seek treatment.

Developing acceptable treatment options has been difficult. Early attempts included cosmetic cover-up, skin grafting, radiation, dermabrasion, cryosurgery, tattooing and electrotherapy but none of these modalities provided cosmetically acceptable results. The development of lasers and their ability to selectively target PWS blood vessels offered an improved treatment option. The pulsed-dye laser (PDL) produces the best results with the lowest incidence of adverse effects. However, the degree of PWS blanching following PDL therapy is variable and unpredictable, and many patients do not achieve complete blanching, even after multiple treatments (5–30 or more). One factor limiting therapeutic efficacy may be the inability of PDL to destroy microvessels (diameter (D) < 20 μm), which may contribute significantly to the clinical appearance of PWS lesions. Because of the limited patient response to current therapy, alternative treatment approaches should be explored.

Hemangiomas are proliferative vascular lesions that generally present at birth or shortly thereafter and grow rapidly during the first months of life. Hemangiomas generally regress with time, and as such, treatment of these lesions is controversial and generally reserved for lesions that are rapidly growing, problematic because of ulceration, bleeding or secondary infection, or impinging on vital structures such as the eyes or nose. Treatment options include intralesional or systemic steroids, PDL therapy, and interferon. Each of these options has risks, some significant, and lesion clearing without scarring is often difficult to achieve. Therefore, alternative treatment options for hemangiomas should also be explored.

Despite the demonstrated propensity of PDT to destroy the tumor vascular compartment and the potential to remove vessels of varied size, PDT has been applied only rarely for treatment of vascular lesions including PWSs and hemangiomas. Careful selection of photosensitizer and wavelength for light irradiation is required for successful implementation of PDT as a treatment of vascular lesions, so that injury may be localized to vessels at a desired depth, allowing effective treatment without significant damage to the overlying skin.

An ideal photosensitizer for PDT treatment of vascular lesions would have the following characteristics: 1) vascular compartmentalization; 2) proven safety and efficacy in humans; and 3) photosensitivity of relatively short duration. While topical ALA-PDT has been considered by some for treatment of vascular lesions, the current authors believe this approach is unlikely to result in significant success. Though there certainly is proven safety and efficacy in humans and a short duration of photosensitivity, there is no vehicle at present which will allow epidermal penetration and subsequent vascular compartmentalization.

Wang et al actually demonstrated increased blood flow rather than vascular sludging or occlusion immediately after topical ALA-PDT treatment of nonmelanoma skin cancers. This increased perfusion persisted in many of the lesions at a 1-week post-treatment follow-up visit, and was thought to represent an inflammatory reaction. It is possible that irradiation and light doses significant enough to cause vascular injury could be achieved, but such parameters would result in significant epidermal destruction, which is unlikely to lead to an acceptable cosmetic result.

Systemic ALA-PDT was utilized in a recent pilot study for vascular lesion treatment. Evans and Kurwa used orally administered ALA (30 mg/kg) and PDT to treat patients with PWS. Each lesion was divided into three equal areas, which were treated with (1) PDL alone (1.5 ms; 6.5 J/cm^2), (2) PDL 1 h after administration of 5-ALA, or (3) PDL 2 h after administration of 5-ALA. Patients received three treatments at four weekly intervals. No significant difference was found between the three treatment areas. Several factors may have contributed to the results. The relatively short pulse duration of the PDL (1.5 ms) may not allow adequate generation of cytotoxic species to achieve prolonged vascular effect. Moreover, while systemic administration of ALA will increase exposure of the vascular endothelial cells to the drug and presumably the light-induced photochemical reaction, currently available forms of ALA are not vascular specific making it difficult to find optimal treatment parameters which will allow selective and significant vascular destruction without epidermal injury.

Kelly et al have demonstrated that PDT may be a good treatment option for vascular lesions either alone or in combination with other therapies. However, at this time, there is no optimal formulation of ALA for this indication and as such, other photosensitizers such as benzoporphyrin derivative monoacid ring A or hematoporphyrin derivatives may be preferred choices. In unpublished pilot studies on non-facial PWS of adults, porfimer sodium PDT achieved good PWS blanching, but significant epidermal disruption occurred (J.S. Nelson, M.D., Ph.D, personal communication). Superficial and deep vasculature are affected by PDT and as such, treatment must be approached cautiously. Further studies are needed to clarify dosing and treatment regimens, and to maximize safety.

Conclusion

ALA-PDT has been attempted for a wide range of dermatologic entities other than the commonly utilized indications of actinic keratoses, acne, basal cell carcinoma and squamous cell carcinoma. ALA-PDT treatment of cutaneous T-cell lymphoma has been demonstrated to be successful in several studies and is a reasonable treatment alternative especially for difficult-to-treat lesions; however parameter optimization is required. Treatment of psoriasis, lichen sclerosus, lichen planus and scleroderma may be useful, but treatment tolerability needs to be improved and treatment strategy further investigated. ALA-PDT treatment of vascular lesions has also been implemented, but since current delivery formulations are likely to limit the success of this approach, new photosensitizers and regimens need to be tested.

Acknowledgments

We would like to gratefully acknowledge the assistance of Drs Genady Kostenich and Sol Kimel during preparation of this chapter.

Further Reading

Bissonnette R, Tremblay J, Juzenas P et al 2002 Systemic photodynamic therapy with aminolevulinic acid induces apoptosis in lesional T cell lymphocytes of psoriatic plaques. Journal of Investigative Dermatology 119:77–83 (Treatment of psoriasis with oral ALA [varying dosage and absorption time] and blue light with post-treatment biopsies demonstrating T cell lymphocyte apoptosis)

Boehncke W-H, Konig K, Ruck A et al 1994 In vitro and in vivo effects of photodynamic therapy in cutaneous T cell lymphoma. Acta Dermatologica Venereologica 74:201–205 (In vivo fluorescence was used to document the ability of PDT to inhibit proliferation of malignant T cells)

Boehnke W, Sterry W, Kaufmann R 1994 Treatment of psoriasis by topical photodynamic light therapy with polychromatic light. Lancet 343:801 (Treatment of psoriasis with topical ALA and polychromatic light compared to contralateral plaques treated with dithranol)

Collins P, Robinson D, Stringer M, Stables G, Sheehan-Dare R 1997 The variable response of plaque psoriasis after a single treatment with topical 5-aminolevulenic acid photodynamic therapy. British Journal of Dermatology 137:743–749 (Treatment of psoriasis with one treatment of topical ALA and polychromatic light)

Coors EA, von den Driesch P 2004 Topical photodynamic therapy for patients with therapy-resistant lesions of cutaneous T-cell lymphoma. Journal of the American Academy of Dermatology 50:363–367 (Evaluated treatment of resistant cutaneous T-cell lymphoma lesions with topical ALA-PDT)

Edstrom DW, Porwit A, Ros A-M 2001 Photodynamic therapy with topical 5-aminolevulenic acid for mycosis fungoides: clinical and histological response. Acta Dermatologica Venereologica 81:184–188 (Evaluation of 5-ALA-PDT for treatment of plaque and tumor lesions of mycosis fungoides)

Evans AV, Kurwa HA 2004 Treatment of port wine stains using photodynamic therapy with systemic 5-aminolaevulinic acid as an adjunct to pulsed dye laser therapy. Lasers in Surgery and Medicine S16:19 (Evaluation of PWS blanching after treatment with oral ALA and PDL compared to PDL therapy alone)

Fritsch C, Lehmann P, Stahl W et al 1998 Optimum porphyrin accumulation in epithelial skin tumours and psoriatic lesions after topical application of delta-aminolaevulinic acid. British Journal of Cancer 79:1603–1608 (Evaluates the time course of porphyrin metabolite formation after topical application of delta-aminolevulinic acid to epithelial skin tumors and psoriasis, in order to determine the optimal application time)

Hillemanns P, Untch M, Prove F et al 1999 Photodynamic therapy of vulvar lichen sclerosis with 5-aminolevulenic acid. Obstetrics & Gynecology 93:71–74 (Pilot study demonstrating symptomatic improvement of vulvar lichen sclerosis for up to 6 months after ALA-PDT therapy)

Ibbotson SH 2002 Topical 5-aminolevulinic acid photodynamic therapy for the treatment of skin conditions other than non-melanoma skin cancer. British Journal of Dermatology 146:178–188 (Review of the use of topical ALA-PDT for treatment of skin conditions other than non-melanoma skin cancers)

Karrer S, Abels C, Landthaler M, Szeimies R 2000 Topical photodynamic therapy for localized scleroderma. Acta Dermatologica Venereologica 80:26–27 (Localized scleroderma lesions show qualitative and quantitative improvement with ALA-PDT therapy)

Karrer S, Bosserhoff A, Weiderer P et al 2003 Influence of 5-aminolevulenic acid and red light on collagen metabolism in human dermal fibroblasts. Journal of Investigative Dermatology 120:325–331 (Fibroblasts show increased production of collagenase mRNA and type I collagen mRNA after ALA-PDT)

Kelly KM, Kimel S, Smith T et al 2004 Combined photodynamic and photothermal induced injury enhances damage to in vivo model blood vessels. Lasers in Surgery and Medicine 34:407–413 (Evaluation of vascular effects after combined PDT plus PDL as compared to PDT alone or PDL alone in a chick chorioallantoic model)

Kirby B, Whitehurst C, Moore JV, Yates VM 1999 Treatment of lichen planus of the penis with photodynamic therapy. British Journal of Dermatology 141:765–766 (Case report of penile hypertrophic lichen planus resolved after 2 treatments of ALA-PDT)

Leman JA, Dick DC, Morton CA 2002 Topical 5-ALA photodynamic therapy for the treatment of cutaneous T-cell lymphoma. Clinical and Experimental Dermatology 27:516–518 (Case report of topical ALA-PDT for plaque stage cutaneous T-cell lymphoma)

Markham T, Sheehan K, Collins P 2001 Topical 5-aminolaevulinic acid photodynamic therapy for tumour-stage mycosis fungoides. British Journal of Dermatology 144:1262 (Case report of topical ALA-PDT for tumor stage mycosis fungoides)

Morton CA, Brown SB, Collins S et al 2002 Guidelines for topical photodynamic therapy: report of a workshop of the British photodermatology group. British Journal of Dermatology 146:552–567 (Review of topical PDT for treatment of dermatologic disease)

Orenstein A, Haik J, Tamir J et al 2000 Photodynamic therapy of cutaneous lymphoma using 5-aminolevulinic acid topical application. Dermatologic Surgery 26:765–770 (Evaluation of PP accumulation and results of ALA-PDT treatment in patients with cutaneous T-cell lymphoma)

Oseroff AR, Whitaker J, Conti C et al 1996 Effects of fluence and intensity in PDT of cutaneous T-cell lymphoma with topical ALA: High intensities spare the epidermis. Journal of Investigative Dermatology 100:602 (An abstract evaluating the efficacy and epidermal toxicity of ALA-PDT for cutaneous T-cell lymphoma)

Pagliaro J, Elliott T, Bulsara M et al 2004 Cold air photodynamic therapy of basal cell carcinomas and Bowen's disease: an effective addition to treatment: a pilot study. Dermatologic Surgery 30:63–66 (Evaluated the use of cold air analgesia during PDT for superficial skin malignancies)

Robinson D, Collins P, Stringer M et al 1999 Improved response of plaque psoriasis after multiple treatments with topical 5-delta aminolevulinic acid photodynamic therapy. Acta Dermatologica Venereologica 79:451–455 (Multiple treatments of psoriasis with topical ALA and polychromatic light)

Stringer M, Collins P, Robinson D et al 1996 The accumulation of protoporphyrin IX in plaque psoriasis after topical application of 5-aminolevulinic acid indicates a potential for superficial photodynamic therapy. Journal of Investigative Dermatology 107:76–81 (Psoriatic plaques show increased fluorescence after topical 5-ALA application)

Wang I, Andersson-Engels S, Nilsson GE et al 1997 Superficial blood flow following photodynamic therapy of malignant non-melanoma skin tumours measured by laser Doppler perfusion imaging. British Journal of Dermatology 136:184–189 (Evaluation of blood flow dynamics during and after treatment of non-melanoma skin tumors with topical ALA-PDT)

Wang I, Bauer B, Andersson-Engels S 1999 Photodynamic therapy utilizing topical δ-aminolevulinic acid in non-melanoma skin malignancies of the eyelid and the periocular skin. Acta Ophthalmologica Scandinavica 77:182–188 (Evaluated the use of topical ALA-PDT for peri-ocular skin malignancies)

Weinstein G, McCullough J, Jeffes E et al 1994 Photodynamic therapy (PDT) of psoriasis with topical delta aminolevulinic acid (ALA): a pilot dose-ranging study. Photodermatology, Photoimmunology, and Photomedicine 10:92. (Treatment of psoriasis with varying concentrations of topical ALA and UVA)

Skin Rejuvenation

8

Jaggi Rao, Mitchel P. Goldman, Michael H. Gold

Introduction

The problem being treated

Chronic sun exposure results in characteristic cutaneous changes that are challenging to treat. The signs of cumulative photodamage, also known as dermatoheliosis or photoaging, include wrinkling, irregular thinning of the epidermis, blotchy hyperpigmentation, telangiectasia formation, and the development of premalignant actinic keratoses (AKs). Most commonly afflicting the facial skin, these changes may occur in any photodistributed anatomic site.

This chapter will describe in detail how to utilize photodynamic therapy (PDT) with topical 5-aminolevulinic acid (ALA) and various coherent and noncoherent light sources to effectively improve the different components of photodamaged skin. In addition to achieving an improved cosmetic appearance, photorejuvenation with PDT-ALA (as detailed in other chapters in this text) is capable of treating AKs to prevent their possible progression to squamous cell carcinomas (SCCs) as well as superficial basal cell carcinoma (BCC) and even dystrophic pigmented lesions.

Etiology and Nature of Photoaging

Since World War II, the socioeconomic influences of outdoor activities have made sun exposure and sun tanning a more desirable way of life, and golden-brown tanned skin has become a symbol of good health, attraction, and affluence. Unfortunately, a dramatic increase in melanomas, nonmelanoma skin cancers, and 'pre-cancers' (AKs and lentigo maligna) has paralleled the increased sun-exposure habit. More visibly, the clinical signs of dermatoheliosis have become increasingly apparent, giving this sun-loving population a prematurely aged appearance. Of all anatomic sites, the head and neck, especially the face, are areas of predilection due to their exposure to the sun.

Past reports have focused on UVB radiation (290–320 nm) as the band of solar radiation responsible for sunburning, dermatoheliosis and skin cancer development. It is now known that concern should be extended to include the UVA spectrum (320–400 nm), which contributes to all of these problems to some degree and with its deeper penetration probably affects collagen and elastin degradation more than UVB.

The histological substrate for dermatoheliosis is solar elastosis. This is seen as a pathological clumping and eventual homogenization and basophilia of the superficial elastic connective tissue of the dermis. The coarseness of skin lines and depth of wrinkles are the clinical manifestations of the focal aggregation of elastotic material. As elastin content increases in the dermis, collagen proportionately decreases. This massive loss in collagen and similar degenerative changes are likely due to metalloproteases and cytokines released by keratinocytes, fibroblasts and inflammatory cells affected by chronic solar radiation. Long-term exposure to solar radiation is also damaging to the microcirculation of the skin. Many vessels are obliterated, reducing cutaneous oxygen supply, establishing hypoxia and functional impairment to surrounding cells. Vessels that survive are variably dilated, resulting in visible erythema and telangiectasias at the skin surface. The normally horizontal vascular plexuses within the dermis are disturbed and often replaced by random tortuous loops.

At the level of the epidermis, photodamaged skin initially demonstrates acanthosis as a result of chronic stimulation. The acanthotic epidermis is accompanied by cellular atypia, loss of keratinocyte polarity and marked irregularities in cell size. It has been shown that keratinocytes from photodamaged skin have a shorter lifespan than those from protected skin, perhaps as a protective mechanism to prevent carcinogenesis. However, if these cellular changes are marked, the clinical result is an actinic keratosis, a premalignant or early cancerous in situ lesion characterized as a red, scaly, well-demarcated papule or macule. Of note, epidermal malignancies such as BCC and SCC arise almost exclusively on actinically damaged skin. In end-stage photoaging, patchy epidermal atrophy occurs. This may be the cause for irregular epidermal thinning and the translucent appearance often seen in dermatoheliosis.

Melanocytes increase in size and number with chronic sun exposure, resulting in hyperpigmented macules (solar lentigines and ephelides) and blotchy pigmented patches. With time, cellular atypia of melanocytes may occur, resulting in the formation of a lentigo maligna, widely regarded as a melanoma in situ.

Therapeutic Challenges

The broad term 'rejuvenation' elegantly encompasses treatment of any or all of the characteristic clinical elements of cutaneous photodamage. The term implies a 'reversal' of the photoaging process and connotes a romantic and mythical 'fountain of youth' approach to therapy. In this sense, the name is a misnomer as it is not the photoaging process that is reversed, but rather, it is enhancement of the overall cosmetic appearance through elimination or masking of unwanted dysesthetic components. Nonetheless, the term has solidified itself in the lexicon of cosmetic surgery and is likely to gain even greater popularity as our ever-growing aging population searches for a solution to these undesirable features.

Photorejuvenation describes the use of coherent and noncoherent light-based devices to perform esthetic rejuvenation. This may include several types of vascular and pigment lasers, as well as those that stimulate dermal fibroblasts to produce collagen. More recently, the use of intense pulsed light (IPL) technology has revolutionized photorejuvenation by its ability to address the pigmentary and vascular components of photoaging, and fine wrinkling to a lesser degree. This is all performed with relative ease and efficiency, and minimal downtime.

Several medical and surgical therapeutic modalities exist for the treatment of dermatoheliosis, especially as these changes pertain to the face (See Box 8.1). Most of these treatment options are specific for only one of the characteristic components of photoaging, and fall short of complete rejuvenation. The few remaining therapies that address more than one element do so at the expense of treating each element with less than maximal efficacy. Even IPL as monotherapy for photorejuvenation is not very effective for the treatment of

---

Medical and surgical therapies to reduce the cutaneous signs of photoaging

Medical
Environment
    Eliminate actinic exposure
    Eliminate cigarette smoking and exposure
Topical agents
    Alpha-hydroxy acids
    Beta-hydroxy acids
    Estrogen
    Melatonin
    Retinoids
    Sunscreens (chemical and physical)
    Vitamins C, E
    Green tea extract
    Growth factors (TGF-beta)
Chemical peels
    Alpha- and beta-hydroxy acids, trichloroacetic acid,
        Jessner's, phenol
Injectable agents (includes soft tissue augmentation)
    Autologous fat transplantation
    Botulinum toxin
    Collagen
    Hyaluronic acid
    Polymethylmethacrylate (PMMA), hydroxyapatite,
        Gore-Tex or other permanent implants
    Vein transfer
Hormone replacement therapy
    Estrogen
    Growth hormone

Surgical
Blepharoplasty
Brow-lift
Cervicofacial rhytidectomy (face-lift)
Carbon dioxide or Erbium laser resurfacing
Dermabrasion or microdermabrasion
Laser treatment of telangiectasias (585–595 nm)
Laser treatment of pigment (Q-switched 694 nm, 755 nm,
    1064 nm)
Lasers designed to stimulate collagen production (585 nm,
    1320 nm, 1450 nm)
Intense pulsed light (IPL)
Radiofrequency devices

Box 8.1 Medical and surgical therapies to reduce the cutaneous signs of photoaging

AKs. Until the advent of PDT, rejuvenation with multiple modalities was the best plan for the treatment of photoaging.

A common combination treatment regimen for photodamage with premalignant lesions includes facelift surgery to reduce unwanted wrinkles in association with laser resurfacing and/or chemical peeling for AKs, pigment-specific lasers such as the Q-switched alexandrite or ruby laser or IPL for hyperpigmentation, and vascular lasers or IPL for telangiectasia. Although such combinations may be successful, they are often very costly, time consuming, have results that are largely user dependent, and are associated with periods of downtime that patients dislike. Not uncommonly, side effects such as pigmentary alterations and rarely scarring may also result.

Photorejuvenation with PDT, recently dubbed 'photodynamic photorejuvenation', represents the newest breakthrough in rejuvenation therapy for photoaging. Yielding excellent cosmetic results with acceptable downtime, PDT photorejuvenation is well tolerated, cost efficient and has been shown to improve each of the different components of photodamaged skin.

Patient selection

Fair-skinned individuals are at most risk for photoaging. Pigmented skin is only partially resistant to solar radiation. Even the most darkly pigmented individuals have only about a decade of lag time from their light-skinned counterparts with regard to the development of solar elastosis. Although the microscopic features of dermatoheliosis occur in all races, cutaneous neoplasms are rare in blacks, Asians and east Indians.

Photorejuvenation with PDT is indicated for patients who demonstrate any component of photoaging (wrinkling, irregular thinning of the epidermis, blotchy hyperpigmentation, and telangiectasia formation) with evidence of AKs. In contrast, IPL photorejuvenation alone is able to improve each of the different components of photodamaged skin, except AKs. PDT has been found to be especially useful in patients with multiple AKs that are widespread on the face and scalp. In these cases, a cost analysis has revealed PDT to be more economical (and tolerable) than multiple sessions of cryotherapy.

Of interest, there is growing experience to suggest that PDT photorejuvenation may accelerate the effects of the same treatment with IPL alone, thereby decreasing the number of treatment sessions to achieve the same result. Anecdotal experience suggests that one treatment with ALA–IPL is equivalent to three treatments with IPL alone for improvement in fine wrinkles, pigmentation and vascular ectasia. This implies that PDT enhances the effects of IPL photorejuvenation, and expands the indication to include those photodamaged individuals who do not have premalignant skin lesions.

Expected benefits

A number of peer-reviewed reports have appeared in the medical literature regarding treatment of AKs with ALA-PDT. The results show between 80–100% clearance for AKs (see Box 8.2). Bowen's disease (SCC in-situ), superficial BCCs and SCCs have also been successfully treated with the ALA-PDT combination at slightly lower clearance rates. Significantly, invasive carcinomas, including deep BCCs, and potentially metastatic lesions, such as SCCs, must be treated with caution when using PDT. Larger, definitive studies are required to delineate the appropriate application of PDT for such cancers since clearance of the superficial aspect of the tumors does not necessarily imply total removal of all of the underlying tumors.

In the pivotal Phase III clinical trials that confirmed the usefulness of ALA-PDT for the treatment of nonhyperkeratotic AKs, 243 subjects with between four and 15 nonhyperkeratotic AKs of the face and scalp were randomly assigned to receive 20% 5-ALA plus blue light PDT treatment or vehicle plus blue light therapy. More than 70% of the patients who had one treatment maintained complete clearance of all AKs at 12 weeks. For those patients who were not complete responders, a second ALA-PDT treatment was performed 8 weeks after the initial treatment. At the conclusion of these trials, 88% of the ALA-PDT-treated patients had greater than or equal to 75% response vs. 20% of patients in the vehicle/control group. Side effects associated with the PDT response included stinging, burning, itching, erythema, and edema – all transient, local symptoms confined only to the skin, and were found in both the ALA-PDT and vehicle-PDT groups. Following the procedure, many patients required a 'healing period' lasting up to 1 week. Less than 3% of patients discontinued the light therapy because of these symptoms. Of interest, nearly all (94%) of the patients in these

Recent peer-reviewed reports of ALA–PDT to treat of AKs			
Authors	**Year(s)**	**Sensitizer/light source**	**Results**
Kennedy et al	1990	20% ALA/filtered slide projector	Complete response in 90%
Wolf et al	1993	20% ALA/filtered slide projector	80–100% response
Morton et al	1995	20% ALA/filtered slide projector	80–100% response
Fijan et al	1995	20% ALA/filtered slide projector	80–100% response
Calzavara-Pinton	1995	20% ALA/argon laser	100% response
Szeimies et al	1996	10% ALA/red light	Complete remission in 71%
Jeffes et al	1997	10–30% ALA/argon laser	91% face/scalp; trunk/extremities 45%
Fritsch et al	1998	20% ALA/green light	Painless
Kurwa et al	1999	20% ALA/nonlaser light	More rapid response than 5-fluorouracil/equivalent results at 6 months
Pinzi et al	2000	20% ALA/incoherent light source	100% response
Jeffes et al	2001	20% ALA/blue light	Complete clearance in 88%

Box 8.2 Recent peer-reviewed reports of ALA–PDT to treat of AKs

Phase III clinical trails rated their cosmetic response as good to excellent.

These Phase III clinical trials required that ALA be allowed to incubate on the skin surface for 14–18 h prior to light treatment. Since then, it has been found that the efficacy of a short contact time of 1 h is as efficacious as longer drug applications. This important fact has reformed ALA-PDT by making it a more practical, convenient and comfortable in-office procedure with relatively little patient and downtime. As such, the procedure has been made into a 'single visit per session' treatment modality. This has allowed for expansion in innovation and research by clinicians that have yielded the novel findings described later.

For example, it has been found that cosmetic treatments already being performed by laser surgeons for photorejuvenation and acne vulgaris may be improved by adding ALA-PDT to the therapeutic routines. In a paper reported by Ruiz-Rodriguez et al, 17 patients with varying degrees of photodamage and AKs (a total of 38 lesions) were treated with two sessions of ALA-PDT, each separated by a month, with 4-hour ALA incubation followed by exposure to an IPL light source. A total of 33 of 38 AKs disappeared within 3 months of follow up. The technique was well tolerated and cosmetic results were excellent in all patients.

In a preliminary study by Gold, short contact (30 min to 1 h incubation), full-face 20% 5-ALA solution utilizing IPL was administered to ten patients with significant dermatoheliosis and AKs. Patients received three IPL treatments with ALA-PDT at 1-month intervals and follow-up visits at 1 and 3 months. Over 85% of the targeted AKs responded to this therapy. In addition, 90% of patients achieved a greater than 75% overall improvement compared to baseline. Improvement in crow's feet and tactile roughness were seen in all patients. Of the study participants, 90% showed improvement in mottled hyperpigmentation and 50% in facial erythema.

The pulsed-dye laser (PDL) has also been found to be effective in treating AKs and photodamage in combination with ALA. Alexiades-Armenakas et al reported on the use of a 585 nm vascular laser 3–18 h after ALA application in 35 patients. The group evaluated 2561 face and scalp AKs with clearances noted at 99.9% at 10 d, 98.4% at 2 months, and 90.1% at 4 months. Lesions on the extremities showed a 61.4% response rate at 10 d and 49.1% at 2 months. Torso lesions responded at 54.5% at 10 d and 74.4% at 2 months. The authors concluded that by using nonpurpuric parameters for the PDL, safe and high efficacy rates could be obtained with minimal discomfort, rapid treatment and recovery times, as well as excellent cosmetic outcomes.

Goldman et al studied 32 patients with moderate photodamage and multiple AKs utilizing short contact (1 h drug incubation), full-face ALA and blue light therapy (a single treatment). At the end of the 6-month clinical trial, lesion counts revealed a 90% clearance of the AKs. There was also an improvement in skin texture in 72% and skin pigmentation in 59%. Of note, 62.5% of his patients found this therapy less painful than cryotherapy.

These results show the potential utility of a variety of coherent and noncoherent light sources in improving AKs and the features of photorejuvenation by utilizing short-contact, full-face ALA-PDT. IPL and laser therapies, both fairly common in many offices already, may be enhanced by the addition of ALA-PDT. As well as treating multiple AKs, nonmelanoma skin cancer, and the clinical effects of photodamage, it is possible that cosmetic photorejuvenation treatments with ALA-PDT may prevent or delay the onset of nonmelanoma skin cancers.

A recent cost analysis for the treatment of AKs performed by the British Photodermatology Group found ALA-PDT to be less expensive than cryotherapy (£119 vs. £160, respectively) with comparable clearance projections but lower 'complication' costs to cover ulceration and/or infection. Further, the Group found the cost of topical 5-fluorouracil therapy to be £171 with higher recurrence and complication rates. This suggests that in addition to the convenience, comfort and tolerability of ALA-PDT, it is also an economically superior modality for photorejuvenation.

Overview of Treatment Strategy

Treatment approach

The use of PDT in dermatology has great promise due to the fact that an appropriate photosensitizer or precursor of the photosensitizer can be accumulated selectively in either dystrophic skin cells or sebaceous glands. With exposure to a light source of an appropriate wavelength, the sensitizer will produce activated oxygen species, and/or singlet oxygen radicals, which are cytotoxic to the cells containing them. A variety of cutaneous malignancies and other entities, such as AKs and acne vulgaris, have been treated successfully with PDT over the past several years.

In 1990, ALA was introduced as a new photosensitizing agent. This 'prodrug' is a photosensitizer with the ability to penetrate through the stratum corneum to ultimately collect into a variety of dystrophic skin cells and tumors, as well as sebaceous glands. Once ALA collects within these cells, it is transformed into protoporphyrin IX (PpIX), a highly photoactive porphyrin derivative that is involved in the endogenous heme biosynthetic pathway (see Fig. 8.1). PpIX can most readily be activated by either a red or blue light source to achieve tissue destruction through the release of activated oxygen species. The absorption spectrum for porphyrin is shown in Figure 8.2.

After an appropriate incubation period (now thought to be 30–60 min), ALA may be activated by a variety of lasers and light sources. These include blue light (405–420 nm), red light (635 nm), PDLs (585–595 nm), and intense pulsed-light sources (500–1200 nm). All of these devices have shown comparable safety and efficacy in PDT and can be utilized for photorejuvenation.

Patient interviews

Patients who are seeking photorejuvenation with PDT should be assessed for a good general health status, absence of photosensitivity disorders and freedom from potentially photosensitizing medications. They should demonstrate any or all of the components of dermatoheliosis. Lastly, they should be capable of understanding pre- and post-treatment care instructions and have the ability to read and sign a written consent for treatment. A sample consent form is presented in Box 8.3.

In general, the treatment strategy is similar for any given patient, with minor considerations. One consideration that the authors have found important is patient gender. This becomes an issue when treating male patients with IPL devices. Specifically, the heat generated from IPL sources has the ability to depilate hair, in this case, follicles of the beard and moustache region. In addition, the presence of large hair follicles can cause the patient greater discomfort due to transmission of heat energy to underlying tissues that may possess greater innervation. For these reasons, the authors refrain from treating beard regions in males with IPL, instead preferring to use either blue light or PDLs on these areas.

Treatment techniques
Patients

Photodynamic photorejuvenation is ideal for patients with signs of chronic sun damage. The relevant features of such damage are wrinkling, irregular thinning of the epidermis, blotchy hyperpigmentation, telangiectasia formation, and the development of premalignant AKs (see Fig. 8.1). Current

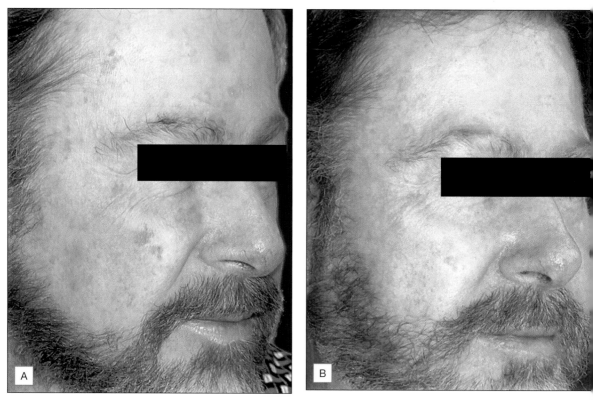

Fig. 8.1 Before and after photodynamic therapy in the treatment of AKs

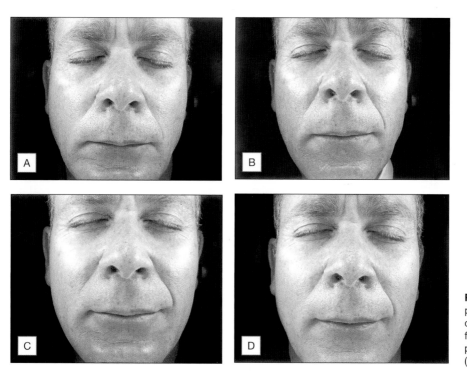

Fig. 8.2 The temporal progression and resolution of the transient side effects from photodynamic photorejuvenation. (**A**) Pre (**B**) Day 1 (**C**) Day 2 (**D**) Day

---

Sample patient consent form

Client consent for Levulan PDT

Levulan (aminolevulinic acid 20%) is a naturally occurring photosensitizing compound which has been approved by the FDA to treat pre-cancerous skin lesions called AK. Levulan is applied to the skin and subsequently 'activated' by specific wavelengths of light. This process of activating Levulan with light is termed PDT. The purpose of activating the Levulan is to improve the appearance and reduce acne rosacea, acne vulgaris, sebaceous hyperplasia, decrease oiliness of the skin, and improve texture and smoothness by minimizing pore size. Any pre-cancerous lesions are also simultaneously treated. The improvement of these skin conditions (other than AK) is considered an 'off-label' use of Levulan.

I understand that Levulan will be applied to my skin for 30–60 minutes. Subsequently, the area will be treated with a specific wavelength of light to activate the Levulan. Following my treatment, I must wash off any Levulan on my skin. I understand that I should avoid direct sunlight for 24 hours following the treatment due to photosensitivity. I understand that I am not pregnant.

Anticipated side effects of Levulan treatment include discomfort, burning, swelling, redness and possible skin peeling, especially in any areas of sun damaged skin and pre-cancers of the skin, as well as lightening or darkening of skin tone and spots, and possible hair removal. The peeling may last many days, and the redness for several weeks if I have an exuberant response to treatment.

I consent to the taking of photographs of my face before each treatment session. I understand that I may require several treatment sessions spaced 2–4 weeks apart to achieve optimal results.

I understand that medicine is not an exact science, and that there can be no guarantees of my results. I am aware that while some individuals have fabulous results, it is possible that these treatments will not work for me. I understand that alternative treatments include topical medications, oral medications, cryosurgery, excisional surgery, and doing nothing.

I have read the above information and understand it. My questions have been answered satisfactorily by the doctor and his staff. I accept the risks and complications of the procedure. By signing this consent form I agree to have one or more Levulan treatments.

_____
Signature

_____
Print name

_____   _____
Date   Witness

Box 8.3 Sample patient consent form

---

guidelines are based on experience derived from treating Caucasian patients, who are more likely to develop photoaging earlier than darker-skinned individuals. Recent experiences in those with Asian skin have led to similar guidelines. Typically these patients are in otherwise good health with no known contact allergies to ALA, and no photosensitivity disorders. In particular, patients who have any form of porphyria, connective tissue disease, solar urticaria or polymorphous light eruption should be excluded from treatment, for fear of symptom exacerbation. It is good practice to also withhold PDT from patients taking known systemic photosensitizing medications. Examples of these are listed in Box 8.4. Lastly, as the administration of ALA causes photosensitivity for several hours, patients must be judged by the caregiver to comply with post-treatment instructions, especially strict sun avoidance for 24 h.

Equipment

Photosensitizers

In the USA, 20% 5-ALA is available as Levulan Kerastick (DUSA Pharmaceuticals, Wilmington, MA). It is a 20% weight/volume ALA solution with 48% ethanol. The Kerastick has a dermatologic applicator at one end for accurate application of the solution. The applicator tip is attached to flexible plastic tubing with two glass vials. One of the vials contains the ALA in the powder form and the other

Common photosensitizing systemic medications

Antihistamines

Astemizole	Cyclizine	Hydroxyzine	Pyrilamine
Azatadine	Cyproheptadine	Meclizine	Terfenadine
Brompheniramine	Dexchlorpheniramine	Methapyrilene	Trimeprazine
Buclizine	Dimenhydrinate	Methdilazine	Tripelennamine
Carbinoxamine	Diphenhydramine	Orphenadrine	Tripolidine
Chlorpheniramine	Diphenylpyraline	Pheniramine	
Clemastine	Doxylamine	Promethazine	

Contraceptives, oral & estrogens (birth control pills, female sex hormones)

Chlorotrianisene	Estradiol	Ethinyl estradiol	Norethindrone
Diethylstilbestrol	Estrogens, conjugated	Medroxyprogesterone	Norgestrel
Estopipate	Estrogens, esterified	Megestrol	Quinestrol

NSAIDs (antiarthritics)

Diclofenac	Flurbiprofen	Meclofenamate	Piroxicam
Diflunisal	Ibuprofen	Naproxen	Suprofen
Fenoprofen	Ketoprofen	Phenylbutazone	Tolmetin

Phenothiazines (major tranquilizers, anti-emetics)

Acetophenazine	Mesoridazine	Prochlororperazine	Thioridazine
Butaperazine	Methdilazine	Promazine	Trifluoperazine
Carphenazine	Methotrimeprazine	Promethazine	Triflupromazine
Chlorpromazine	Methozsalen	Propiomazine	Trimeprazine
Ethoproprazine	Perphenazine	Psoralens	Triozsalen
Fluphenazine	Piperacetazine	Thiethylperazine	

Sulfonamides ('sulfa' drugs, antimicrobials, anti-infectives)

Acetazolamide	Sulfadoxine	Sulfapyrazone
Sulfacytine	Sulfamethizole	Sulfasalazine
Sulfadiazine	Sulfamethoxazole	Sulfisoxazole

Sulfonylureas (oral anti-diabetics, hypoglycemics)

Acetohexamide	Glipizide	Tolazamide
Chlorpropamide	Glyburide	Tolbutamide

Thiazide diuretics ('water-pills')

Bendroflumethiazide	Chlorothiazide	Hydroflumethiazide	Ploythiazide
Benzthiazide	Cyclothiazide	Methyclothiazide	Trichlormethiazide
Chlorothalidone	Hydrochlorothiazide		

Tetracyclines (antibiotics, anti-infectives)

Chlortetracycline	Doxycycline	Oxytetracycline
Demeclocycline	Minocycline	Tetracycline

Tricyclic antidepressants

Amitriptyline	Desipramine	Imipramine	Protyiptyline
Amoxapine	Doxepin	Nortriptyline	Trimipramine

Herbal supplements

Gingko Biloba	St. John's Wort

Derived from: Medications that Increase Sensitivity to Light: A 1990 Listing, prepared by Jerome I. Levine, 12/90, US Dept of Health & Human Services, FDA 91-8280

Box 8.4 Common photosensitizing systemic medications

vial contains the ethanol solvent. The vials are broken by light manual pressure to the tubing and the contents mixed by rotating the contents back and forth for several minutes. The mixture is then ready for application.

In Europe, a cream formulation is available known as Metvix (PhotoCure ASA, Norway), which is the methyl ester of ALA. The European approval is for the treatment of nonhyperkeratotic AKs of the face and scalp and for BCCs unsuitable for conventional therapy. Recent reports have shown improvements in AKs (70–90%) and superficial BCCs (up to 97% response rate). Cosmetic improvement was also noted. The methyl ester cream of ALA is not yet available in the USA.

Systemic photosensitizers also exist but are not regularly used for skin cancers and other cutaneous lesions.

Light sources

The following are suggested treatment parameters for various coherent and noncoherent light systems for PDT photorejuvenation:

1. IPL Quantum SR (Lumenis Ltd., Yokneam, Israel)
   - 560 nm filter, double-pulse (3.0 ms and 6.0 ms), 20 ms delay, 25–30 J/cm^2, single pass with no overlap
2. Lumenis One (Lumenis Ltd., Yokneam, Israel)
   - 560 nm filter, double-pulse (4.0 ms and 4.0 ms), 20 ms delay, 15–25 J/cm^2, single pass with no overlap
3. Vasculight SR (Lumenis Ltd., Yokneam, Israel)
   - 560 nm filter, double-pulse (3.0 ms and 6.0 ms), 20 ms delay, 30–35 J/cm^2, single pass with no overlap
4. Estelux Pulsed Light System (Palomar Medical Technologies, Burlington, MA)
   - 20 ms, 19–30 J/cm^2, single pass with no overlap
5. Photogenica V Star (Cynosure, Inc., Chelmsford, MA)
   - 585 nm or 595 nm wavelength PDL
   - 10 mm spot size, 40 ms pulse duration, 7.5 J/cm^2, two passes with 50% overlap
6. VBeam (Candela Corporation, Wayland, MA)
   - 595 nm PDL
   - 10 mm spot size, 6 ms pulse duration, 7.5 J/cm^2, two passes with 50% overlap
7. ClearLight (Lumenis Ltd., Yokneam, Israel)
   - 405–420 nm blue light
   - 8–10 min
8. SkinStation (Radiancy, Orangeburg, NY)
   - 500–1200 nm
   - 2 passes, 45 J/cm^2
9. BLU-U (DUSA Pharmaceuticals, Wilmington, MA)
   - Blue light illuminator (peak wavelength 417 nm ± 5 nm)
   - 10–15 min

Treatment algorithm

In the original clinical protocols with the Levulan Kerastick for AKs, the solution was applied to individually identified AKs. Once the solution dried, a second application was applied. The ALA was then allowed to incubate on the skin surface for 14–18 h before the areas to be treated were exposed to visible blue light of 417 nm wavelength. The duration of light exposure was 1000 s with a fluence of 10 J/cm^2. A second treatment would be used 8 weeks later for those lesions that had not responded.

Although these original protocols demonstrated success in treating AKs, the long duration of ALA application, pain during treatment and subsequent downtime limited its attraction for patients and impaired its use as a regular day-to-day procedure. Newer trials have focused primarily on the use of topical 20% 5-ALA solution and have included the broad application of the ALA solution over the entire face, scalp, chest and/or back followed by exposure to the original blue light source, a variety of vascular wavelength laser systems in the 585–600 nm range, and IPL sources in the 550–1200 nm wavelength range. Additionally, shorter incubation times (30 min to 1 h) have been routinely employed to help make the procedures more accessible to patients, reducing the number of clinical visits to 1 d instead of 2 d. The shorter duration of application has made ALA-PDT therapy more tolerable to patients by lessening the potential adverse effect profile, especially minimizing pain and downtime.

The following is a treatment and post-treatment algorithm utilized by the authors. By carefully following this sequence of events and strictly adhering to the methodology described, their patients have been successfully treated by photodynamic photorejuvenation with minimal side effects and near uniform patient satisfaction. Clinical pearls from the authors are italicized. The ALA used in this protocol is Levulan Kerastick (DUSA Pharmaceuticals, Wilmington, MA).

Treatment protocol

1. Patients who have a history of recurring cold sores may start oral Valtrex 500 mg or Famvir 250 mg, two tablets twice daily for 3 d starting on the morning of the PDT session.
2. The patient should gently wash their skin with soap and water. Cetaphil cleanser or a similar cleanser is usually used.
3. The skin should be vigorously scrubbed with acetone prior to ALA application. Acetone scrubbing serves not only to cleanse the skin, but also to increase the penetration of ALA greater than that of isopropyl alcohol pre-treatment. Alternatively or in conjunction with acetone scrubbing, microdermabrasion may be performed to abrade the stratum corneum, which will also enhance penetration of ALA.
4. The two glass ampules in the Kerastick should be broken as per the labeling instructions on the stick. Vigorous shaking of the stick for about 2 min should follow. Shaking serves to mix the ALA powder with the solvent.
5. Levulan, now in liquid form, should be applied to the desired area of treatment by painting the solution on the entire area from the applicator end of the Kerastick. It is recommended that two coats of the solution be applied in any given area to ensure adequate surface ALA for penetration. Additional ALA may be 'spot' treated on AKs for this reason.

   When treating the face, the authors have found it important to get close to the eyes, as it will be apparent that the periorbital skin was not adequately treated otherwise. Care should be taken to avoid the eyelids, cornea and ocular canthi. As a general rule, the volume of ALA in one Kerastick should be sufficient to adequately treat the entire facial skin. Additional sticks should be employed to treat extended sites such as the neck, scalp, chest or limbs.

6. For photorejuvenation, Levulan should incubate for a minimum of 60 min (1 h) while the patient remains indoors, away from direct or reflected sunlight. *Sun avoidance during this period is crucial, as premature and uncontrolled activation of ALA will invariably result in a phototoxic eruption.*
7. After incubation, Levulan should be gently washed from the face with soap and water to remove any surface ALA that may be subsequently activated by PDT. Remnant ALA on the surface of the skin during exposure to an activating light source can result in superficial burning of the epidermis and associated pain, vesiculation and ulceration.
8. Levulan should then be activated by an appropriate light source as per the parameters listed earlier. Appropriate patient and operator eyewear should be used, as per the safety guidelines of the device utilized.

Post-treatment considerations

1. After light exposure, the treated area may respond by demonstrating some erythema and edema. The patient may experience mild symptoms of burning and tingling. These may be reduced and relieved by the immediate application of ice or cold packs. This will help keep the area cool and alleviate any discomfort, as well as decrease swelling. Swelling is most evident around the eyes and is usually more prominent in the morning after treatment.

   During this post-treatment period, PDT-treated skin is very sensitive and may be inflamed, permitting greater penetration of topical agents, which will increase the likelihood of irritant and allergic contact dermatitis. For this reason, the authors advise against the acute use of most topical agents to reduce the 'photodynamic effect.' This includes vitamin E, high-potency corticosteroids, aloe vera, herbal agents and most moisturizers, which may contain potentially irritating and sensitizing preservatives and perfumes. Hydrocortisone 1% may alleviate inflammation without side effects. If the skin becomes dry, hydration may be enhanced by the thin application of petrolatum Aquaphor or Cetaphil moisturizer, which are known to be bland and generally nonirritating. Elevating the head on two pillows when sleeping helps to reduce swelling. Analgesics such as Tylenol or Advil may be taken. The authors also recommend the use of Avene Thermal Spring Water to be applied by the patient liberally during the day. Niadyne skin cleanser and night-time moisturizer is also recommended.

2. Patients must be advised that it is paramount that they avoid direct or reflected sunlight for 24 h after PDT. If this instruction is not strictly followed, phototoxicity is likely to occur. In fact, it is best that patients stay indoors during this period. If this is not possible, outdoor exposure should be very limited, and a physical block

sunscreen of at least SPF 30 should be applied prior to leaving along with a hat, sunglasses and a physical barrier such as a scarf.

Although ALA should be metabolized within a few hours both endogenously and with PDT, the process varies in efficiency according to several patient factors and light source characteristics. As such, a 24-hour safety window is wise to ensure that no photoreactive product is present in the skin to produce adverse reactions. Despite this, some patients remain photosensitive for as long as 40 h after PDT. It should be noted that UVA and visible light readily penetrate through glass, including the windshields of automobiles. Patients should therefore be encouraged to wear physical block sunscreen, a hat, sunglasses and a scarf immediately after treatment, before leaving the office and venturing home. The rationale for a physical block sunscreen is twofold: (1) physical sunscreens are less irritating to inflamed skin, and (2) they work to reflect light, rather than to absorb it, making for a more broad-spectrum sunscreen.

3. With the original 14–18-hour drug incubation period, it was not unusual to take several days for the treated skin to recover from the anticipated photodynamic effect. The area may have been red for 4–6 weeks. Crusting may have occurred after the inflammatory process had settled. Patients may apply make-up once any crusts have healed. On the day after treatment, if scabbing occurs (less than 10% incidence in the original protocol) patients should soak the treated areas with a solution of 1 tsp white vinegar in 1 c of cold water for 20 min every 4–6 h. Ice may be applied directly over the vinegar soaks. The area may be patted dry and hydrocortisone 1% reapplied following the vinegar soaks. With the advent of short-contact, full-face ALA-PDT, a prolonged photodynamic effect is rare. Erythema may last for several days, as indicated, but most patients queried have indicated no associated downtime as a result of this new approach.

If make-up is important to the patient, a mineral-based formulation, such as Jane Iredale Mineral Make-up, which is relatively inert and combines a concealer with sunscreen, is recommended.

4. Patients should be advised that their skin may feel dry and tightened after the second post-procedure day. A good moisturizer should be used daily. Direct sunlight should be avoided for up to 2 weeks, and a minimum SPF 30 sunscreen

should then be used for 4 months. It is good practice to provide patients with an emergency contact number in the event of concerns or complications.

The authors recommend Niadyne moisturizer and Avene Thermal Spring Water.

5. For photodynamic photorejuvenation, a minimum of 2–4 weeks is suggested between subsequent treatment sessions if AKs are present. If these are not present, a 4-week treatment interval is reasonable.

Typically, a series of two to three treatments are needed to most effectively treat AKs. Treatment sessions should never be prescribed in multiple sessions, as it is impossible to predict patient response or side effects after a single session. Instead, sessions should be prescribed on a 'single-treatment basis' upon evaluation at each clinical visit. Maintenance therapy may be required on a yearly basis.

Troubleshooting

It is important that not only the primary caregiver, but also the entire auxiliary and nursing staff involved in the care of the photodynamic photo-rejuvenation patient be knowledgeable about the procedure and respect its potential merits and side effects/complications. Receptionists should be trained on how to manage or direct concerns of pre- and post-treatment patients, and protocols should be instituted to handle any complication in an efficient manner.

Operators of light devices must be thorough with the capabilities of their system and adjust parameters according to the needs and characteristics of their patients. A little time spent to ensure that the treatment is performed appropriately is key to the prevention of future problems.

Side effects, complications and alternative approaches
Side effects

Anticipated side effects of photodynamic photo-rejuvenation with long, 14–18-hour drug incubation include discomfort, burning, swelling, redness and possible skin peeling, especially in areas of sun-damaged skin and AKs. Figure 8.2 demonstrates a series of sequential photographs illustrating the temporal progression and resolution of these effects.

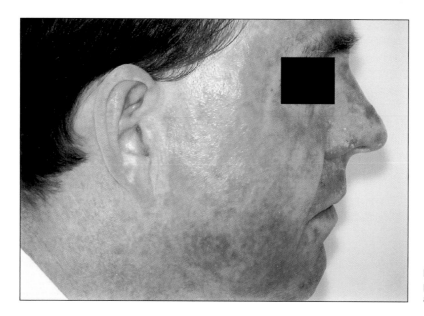

Fig. 8.3 Phototoxic reaction in a patient exposed to sunlight within 24 h after photodynamic photorejuvenation

The peeling may last many days (usually 3–5 d), and the redness for several weeks (usually 1–2 weeks) depending on the intensity of response to treatment. Temporary labial and periorbital swelling may occur, and can last for several days. Moreover, post-inflammatory hyper- and/or hypopigmentation may occur in focal or generalized areas. These are generally temporary and reversible, and more likely in darker skinned individuals. As with IPL therapy, lentigines usually become darker before resolving. Inadvertent hair removal is possible, but this effect is nearly always transient. With the advent of short-contact, full-face ALA-PDT, these photodynamic effects should be minimal. Erythema for 24 h is commonly seen; pain and downtime should be slight.

Complications

The most common complication of photodynamic photorejuvenation is phototoxicity (see Fig. 8.3). In general, this is an exaggerated sunburn. More often than not, this is the result of inadvertent outdoor exposure after PDT, patient underestimation of the likelihood of developing such a reaction and subsequent laxity in following post-treatment instructions, or poor communication on the part of the caregiver to the patient. Phototoxicity is clinically manifested within hours of excess light exposure as intense erythema and edema that is well demarcated within the sites of ALA application. It may be associated with burning pain and hyperesthesia.

The best treatment is prevention through caregiver reinforcement of the need to avoid sun exposure and applying appropriate and frequent sunscreen during the first 24 h after treatment. It is also important to ensure that the patient is not taking medications that can increase cutaneous photosensitivity. Acute treatment of phototoxic reactions includes rest, application of ice, elevation of the affected area to reduce swelling, and time. Topical corticosteroids and moisturizers may offer symptom relief. It is advisable to use ointments over creams and lotions, as ointments have a relatively lower concentration of potentially irritating and sensitizing preservatives and perfumes. The utility of systemic corticosteroids and nonsteroidal anti-inflammatory drugs (NSAIDs) is debatable, and should be evaluated on a case-by-case basis, and only if other forms of intervention fail, by carefully weighing the advantages and disadvantages for a given patient.

The authors have been impressed with the ability of the GentleWaves diode light source as a means to decreasing the phototoxic reaction and subsequent erythema. If possible, the authors have the patient do a 55-second treatment a day or two after the PDT treatment and at weekly intervals.

Cutaneous viral and bacterial infections after photodynamic photorejuvenation are rare, but can occur. Prophylactic antiviral agents in patients with a history of recurrent herpes simplex virus infection or active infection may prevent exacerbation. Thorough patient cleansing of the treated area prior to PDT can prevent superficial bacterial infections such as impetigo and cellulitis. When bacterial infections occur, they are usually at the site of inflammation and erosion of AKs or ALA that has not been adequately washed off the skin surface prior to light treatment. Treatment consists of topical antibiotic preparations such as mupirocin or bacitracin ointment until resolved. Systemic antibiotics are rarely indicated.

Alternate approaches

Alternate forms of ALA other than Levulan have been used, but these formulations are not FDA approved and their use is strongly discouraged for both medical and legal reasons. Because Levulan has been FDA approved since 1999 and therefore maintains strict standards in formulation, its effects are widely known to be safe and predictable. It is not known how long ALA remains stable and active when mixed into a cream or other solution. In addition, it is not known how other 'self-made' ALA creams need to be applied to the skin to achieve an effective concentration in dystrophic cells and/or sebaceous glands. The few cases of allergic contact dermatitis to ALA reported in the literature have been associated with ALA sources in which nonstandardized components have been utilized.

ALA has been formulated in lower concentrations within a unique liposomal delivery system to improve cutaneous penetration. Although this unique preparation has been shown to be very effective in treating AKs, it is not yet a commercially available product and has to be formulated. Because of the very real possibility of phototoxicity, this and other novel formulations of ALA should be left to investigators highly experienced with PDT.

Recalcitrant AKs may represent Bowen's disease lesions (SCC in-situ) or invasive skin cancer, and should be biopsied for histological analysis. As an adjunct to PDT, hyperkeratotic AKs may be additionally treated by traditional therapeutic methods such as cryotherapy, topical 5-fluorouracil, imiquimod and retinoids. Large telangiectasias may be treated with laser devices such as a PDL, 1064 nm Nd:YAG laser, or with a second pass of the IPL at higher fluences and/or pulse durations. The adjuvant use of topical rejuvenative agents including bleaching creams, retinoids, antioxidants and growth factor preparations is currently being studied.

Further Reading

Alexiades-Armenakas M, Bernstein CJ, Chen J, Jacobson L, Geronemus R 2003 Laser-assisted photodynamic therapy of actinic keratoses: long-term follow-up. Journal of Lasers in Surgery and Medicine 15(S):45

Avram DK, Goldman MP 2004 Effectiveness and safety of ALA-IPL in treating actinic keratoses and photodamage. Journal of Drugs in Dermatology 3:S32–S39

Bissonette R, Bergeron A, Liu Y 2004 Large surface photodynamic therapy with aminolevulinic acid: Treatment of actinic keratoses and beyond. Journal of Drugs in Dermatology 3:S26–S31

Calzavara-Pinton PG 1995 Repetitive photodynamic therapy with topical delta-aminolaevulinic acid as an appropriate approach to the routine treatment of superficial non-melanoma skin tumours. [Clinical Trial. Journal Article] Journal of Photochemistry and Photobiology 29(1):53–57

Fijan S, Honigsmann H, Ortel B 1995 Photodynamic therapy of epithelial skin tumours using delta-aminolaevulinic acid and desferrioxamine. British Journal of Dermatology 133:282–288.

Fritsch C, Lang K, Neuse W, Ruzicka T, Lehmann P 1998 Photodynamic diagnosis and therapy in dermatology. Skin Pharmacology Applied Skin Physiology 11:358–373

Gold MH 2002 The evolving role of aminolevulinic acid hydrochloride with photodynamic therapy in photoaging. Cutis 69:8–13

Gold MH 2003 Intense pulsed light therapy for photorejuvenation enhanced with 20% aminolevulinic acid photodynamic therapy. Journal of Lasers in Medicine and Surgery 15(S):47

Goldman MP, Atkin D, Kincad S 2002 PDT/ALA in the treatment of actinic damage: real world experience. Journal of Lasers in Medicine and Surgery 14(S):24

Jeffes EW, McCullough JL, Weinstein GD et al 1997 Photodynamic therapy of actinic keratosis with topical 5-aminolevulinic acid. A pilot dose-ranging study. Archives of Dermatology 133(6):727–732

Jeffes EW, McCullough JL, Weinstein GD, Kaplan R, Glazer SD, Taylor JR 2001 Photodynamic therapy of actinic keratoses with topical aminolevulinic acid hydrochloride and fluorescent blue light. Journal of the American Academy of Dermatology 45(1):96–104

Kaidbey KH, Kligman AM 1979 Acute effect of long wave ultraviolet irradiation on human skin. Journal of Investigative Dermatology 72:253

Kalka K, Merk H, Mukhtar H 2000 Photodynamic therapy in dermatology. Journal of the American Academy of Dermatology 42:389–413

Kennedy JC, Pottier RH, Pross DC et al 1990 Photodynamic therapy with endogenous protoporphyrin IX: basic principles and present clinical experience. Journal of Photochemistry and Photobiology 6:143–148

Kurwa HA, Yong-Gee SA, Seed PT, Markey AC, Barlow RJ 1999 A randomized paired comparison of photodynamic therapy and topical 5-fluorouracil in the treatment of actinic keratoses. Journal of the American Academy of Dermatology 41:414–418

Morton CA, Brown SB, Collins S, et al 2002 Guidelines for topical photodynamic therapy: report of a workshop of the British Photodermatology Group. British Journal of Dermatology 146:552–567

Morton CA, Whitehurst C, Moseley H et al 1995 Development of an alternative light source to lasers for photodynamic therapy: Clinical evaluation in the treatment of pre-malignant non-melanoma skin cancer. Lasers in Medical Science 10:165–171

Osmrod D, Jarvis A 2000 Topical aminolevulinic acid HCl photodynamic therapy. American Journal of Clinical Dermatology 1(2):133–139

Pinzi C, Campolmi P, Moretti S, Guasti A, Rossi R, Cappugi P 2000 Photodynamic therapy for the treatment of primary and secondary (non-melanoma) skin tumours with topical delta-aminolevulinic acid. Giornale Italiano di Dermatologia e Venereologia 135(4):427–431

Ruiz-Rodriguez R, Sanz-Sanchez T, Cordoba S 2002 Photodynamic photorejuvenation. Dermatologic Surgery 28:742–744

Sherris DA, Otley CC, Bartley GB 1998 Comprehensive treatment of the aging face – cutaneous and structural rejuvenation. Mayo Clinic Proceedings 73:139

Szeimies RM, Karrer S, Sauerwald A, Landthaler M 1996 Photodynamic therapy with topical application of 5-aminolevulinic acid in the treatment of actinic keratoses: an initial clinical study. Dermatology 192(3):246–251

Touma D, Whitehead S, Konnikov N, Phillips T, Yaar M, Gilchrist B 2003 Short incubation 8-ALA-PDT for treatment of actinic keratoses and facial photodamage. Journal of Lasers in Medicine and Surgery 15(S):47

Wolf P, Rieger E, Kerl H 1993 An alternative treatment modality for solar keratoses, superficial squamous cell carcinomas and basal cell carcinomas? Journal of the American Academy of Dermatology 28:17–21

Subject Index

Notes

Index entries in **bold** refer to information in tables or boxes: index entries in *italics* refers to figures.

To save space in the index, the following abbreviations have been used:

ALA – 5-aminolevulinic acid
BCC – basal cell carcinoma
IPL – intense pulsed light
MALA – methylaminolevulinic acid
PDT – photodynamic therapy
SCC – squamous cell carcinoma

A

ablative laser vaporization, sebaceous hyperplasia, 9
acanthosis, photoaging, 101
acne, 9
  alternative treatment, 29
  Bruton scale grading, **13**
  causative bacteria, 13, **13**
  IPL, 19
acne PDT, 13–32
  active cooling, 28
  adverse effects, **18,** 29
    erythema, 16
  ALA dose, 23, 28
    stepwise doses, 18
  algorithm, 18–19, 23, *27, 28*
  antibacterial effect, 31–32
  BLU-U PDT, 9
  complications, **18,** 29
    papulopustular lesions, 19, *19*
    'severe reactive acne,' *23*
  equipment, 20–21, 23
    light-emitting diode devices, 21, 23
    metal halide lamps, 21, *27*
  expected benefits, 15–18, *22, 26*
    clinical assessments, **16**
    comedomal lesions, 18
    papulopustular lesion reduction, 15–16, *21*
  indications, 20
  patient interviews, 20
  patient selection, 14–15
  post-hyperpigmentation, 13, *14, 15, 16*
    topical-ALA, 17–18
  reactive acne, 16–17
  systemic ALA, 16–17, 23, 28
    topical ALA *vs.,* 31
  time intervals, 19
  topical ALA, 17–18
    systemic ALA *vs.,* 31
  tretinoin pretreatment, 20, 23
  ultraviolet examination, **14,** *18,* 18–19, *20*

vitamin C iontophoresis, 19, 20, 29
  devices, *30*
  efficacy, *30*
acne rosacea, treatment indications, 20
actinic cheilitis
  histopathology, 34
  PDT clinical trials, 42
actinic keratoses, 7–8, 33–51
  alternative therapies, 49, **50**
  animal models, 54
  clinical presentation, 33–34, *34*
  conventional treatments, 7
  histopathology, 34, *35*
  prevalence, 33
  SCC progression, 7, 33, 34
  see also photoaging
actinic keratoses PDT, 1, 8, 57–62
  active cooling, 60
  advantages, 7–8
  adverse effects, **7,** 8, 44, 49, 59–61 *see also specific effects*
    exuberant reactions, *44*
    hyperpigmentation, 61
    hypopigmentation, 61
  ALA, *6*
    application, 58–59
  algorithm, *45,* 47–49
    active cooling, 49
    drug application, 47, *48*
    IPL, 48
    overnight ALA application, 48
    skin preparation, 47
  benefits, 38–40, 42, *43,* 62, *62*
  BLU-U light source, 35, 45, 47–48, 59
    clinical trials, 39–40
  clinical trials, 38–40
    MALA, 42
  comfort/convenience, 42–43
  complete response rates, 38
  complications, 49
  cost/benefit ratio, 43

actinic keratoses PDT (*cont'd*)
  dosimetry, 35, 36–37
    clinical trials, **39,** 40, 42
    incubation time variation, 37, *37,* 42, 48, 61
  drawbacks, 49–50
  equipment, 46–47
  expected benefits, 103
  future work, 62
  IPL, 10
  Levulan, 8
  lifestyle preferences, 46
  light dose, 35–37, 59
    red light sources, 37
  light sources, 59 *see also individual sources*
    ClearLight source, 35
  long pulse dye laser/IPL, 45–46, *46,* 59
    clinical trials, 40, 42
  major determinants, 44
  MALA, 10, 62
  medical history, 46
  pain control measures, 49, 60
  patient interviews, 46
  patient precautions, 48–49
    concomittant drug therapy, 61
  patient selection, 38, **38,** 57–58
  PpIX concentration, 35
  rationale, 34–35
  session number, 59
  topical ALA formulation, 35
  treatment benefits, **7**
  troubleshooting, 49
active cooling
  acne PDT, 28
  actinic keratoses PDT, 49, 60
  cutaneous T-cell lymphomas PDT, 93
  skin rejuvenation PDT, 110
  warts PDT, 87–88
adverse effects (of PDT), 4
  see also individual effects; individual treatments
alanine transaminase levels, *24*
alkaline phosphatase levels, *24*
5-aminolevulinic acid (ALA), 3–5
  alanine transaminase levels, *24*
  alkaline phosphatase levels, *24*
  aspartate transaminase levels, *24*
  bilirubin levels, *25*
  cholinesterase levels, *25*
  development, 1–2
  dose
    acne PDT, 23, 28
    psoriasis PDT, 94
  gamma glutamyl phosphorylase levels, *25*
  heme biosynthesis, 3
  lactate dehydrogenase levels, *24*
  methyl derivative *see* methylaminolevulinic acid (MALA)
  porphobilinogen formation, 3
  properties, **2**
  skin penetration, 3, 4, *14, 15,* 16, *16*
  structure, *2*
  systemic *vs.* topical, 95, 96
  therapeutic uses, 7–10 *see also individual diseases/
    disorders*
  treatment effects, 3

animal models
  actinic keratoses, 54
  BCC, 55
  SCC, 54–55, *55, 56*
anticoagulant therapy, PDT contraindications, 70
antihistamines, as photosensitizers, **108**
antioxidants
  avoidance post-PDT, 29
  PDT contraindications, 70
antiviral effects (of PDT), 81
application times
  cutaneous T-cell lymphomas PDT, 92
  psoriasis PDT, 94
aspartate transaminase levels, ALA, *24*
aspirin, PDT contraindications, 70

B
basal cell carcinoma (BCC), 8, 53, 65
  conventional treatments, 8
    cryotherapy, 8, 66
    curettage, 8, 66
    cytotoxic agents, 66
    electrodesiccation, 8
    excision, 8, 66
    Mohs' surgery, 8
    PDT *vs.,* **71**
    radiotherapy, 8, 66
  development
    p53 gene, 56
    PTCH gene, 55
  incidence, 53
  morpheaform, 66, *66*
  nodular, 65–66
  pigmented, 66, *66*
  prevention, animal models, 55
basal cell carcinoma (BCC) PDT, 1, 8, 65, *66*
  adverse effects, **7**
  ALA
    adverse effects, **70**
    clinical trials, 68, *68*
    complete clearance rates, 67
    cryosurgery *vs.,* 67
  alternative therapy *vs.,* **71**
  benefits, *68, 69*
  cost analyses, 68
  MALA, 58
    clinical trials, **70**
    complete clearance rates, 67
  nodular, cure rate, 66
  red light penetration, 66
  treatment benefits, **7**
  tumor thickness, 8, 67
benzoporphyrin derivative monoacid ring A, **2, 3**
bilirubin levels, ALA, *25*
blue light PDT, 4
  photorejuvenation, 10
  see also individual types
BLU-U PDT, 4
  acne therapy, 9
  actinic keratoses PDT, 35, 45, 47–48, 59
    clinical trials, 39–40
  protoporphyrin IX activating dose, **5,** *5*

Bowen's disease, 8–9
    adverse effects, **7**
    conventional treatments, 8
    PDT, 8–9, 65, 71–72
        benefits, **7**
        expected benefits, 103
breast cancer metastases, PDT, 65
breastfeeding, PDT contraindications, 78

C

cauterization, sebaceous hyperplasia, 9
chemical peels, actinic keratoses PDT, **50**
chemiluminescent light patches, 5
cholinesterase levels, ALA, *25*
ClearLight source, 4
    acne therapy, 9
    actinic keratoses PDT, 35
clinical trials
    ALA-PDT, BCC, 68, *68*
    dosimetry, actinic keratoses PDT, **39,** 40, 42
    Levulan, 38–39, **39,** 40, *41*
    long pulse dye laser/IPL, 40, 42
    skin rejuvenation, 103–105, **104**
comedomal lesions, acne PDT, 18
complete clearance rates
    actinic keratoses PDT, 38
    BCC ALA-PDT, 67
    BCC MALA-PDT, 67
concomittant drug therapy, actinic keratoses PDT, 61
condyloma acuminata, 71
consent form, skin rejuvenation, *107*
contraceptive drugs, as photosensitizers, **108**
contraindications (to PDT), 70, 78
corticosteroids
    cutaneous T-cell lymphoma therapy, 90
    psoriasis therapy, 94
cosmesis
    skin cancer PDT, 75
    warts PDT, 78
cost analysis
    skin rejuvenation, 105
    warts PDT, 79–81
cryotherapy
    actinic keratoses, 7, 49, **50**
    BCC, 8, 66
        ALA-PDT *vs.,* 67
        PDT *vs.,* **71**
    Bowen's disease, 8
    sebaceous hyperplasia, 9
curettage
    actinic keratoses, 7, 49, **50**
    BCC, 8, 66
        PDT *vs.,* **71**
    Bowen's disease, 8
cutaneous T-cell lymphomas, 89–90
cutaneous T-cell lymphomas, PDT, 65, 89–94, *90,* **91**
    active cooling, 93
    benefits, 90, 92
    nodular, *90*
    patient selection, 90
    side effects/complications, 93
    techniques, 92–93
        in vivo fluorescence monitoring, 92, *92, 93*

cytostatic drugs, PDT contraindications, 70
cytotoxic agents, BCC, 66

D

dermatoheliosis, 101
desferrioxamine, as penetration enhancer, 72
desquamation, post-PDT, 44, 49

E

edema
    actinic keratoses, 44, 49, 60
    photorejuvenation, 112
    skin cancer, 74–75
EDTA, as penetration enhancer, 72
electrocautery, Bowen's disease, 8
electrodessication, BCC, 8
emission spectrum
    light-emitting diodes, *28*
    metal halide lamps, *27*
energy density
    light-emitting diodes, *28*
    metal halide lamps, *28*
erythema
    acne PDT, 16, 29
    actinic keratoses PDT, 42–43, 44, 60, 61
    photorejuvenation PDT, 112
    skin cancer PDT, 74–75
ethnicity, ALA skin penetration, 3
evolution (of PDT), 1
excision surgery
    actinic keratoses PDT, **50**
    BCC, 8, 66
        PDT *vs.,* **71**
excitation spectrum, protoporphyrin IX (PpIX), 20
expected benefits (of PDT), 5

F

Fitzpatrick skin types, **33**
5-fluorouracil, actinic keratoses, 7, 49
folliculitis, treatment indications, 20
fractionation, cutaneous T-cell lymphomas PDT, 92

G

gamma glutamyl phosphorylase levels, ALA, *25*
Gorlin's syndrome, 58

H

health insurance exclusion, warts PDT, 80–81
hemangiomas, 97
hematoporphyrin, 1
heme biosynthesis, ALA, 3
herbal supplements, as photosensitizers, **108**
2-[1-hexyloxyethyl]-2-devinyl pyrophorbide-a, **2**
human papilloma virus (HPV), 77–88
    etiology, 77
    see also warts
hyperpigmentation
    actinic keratoses PDT, 61
    post-acne PDT, 13, *14, 15, 16,* 17–18
    psoriasis PDT, 96
    skin rejuvenation, 112
    warts PDT, 78–79

hypopigmentation
    actinic keratoses PDT, 61
    skin rejuvenation, 112

I

immune modifiers, actinic keratoses PDT, **50**
immunosuppression, psoriasis therapy, 94
infections, skin rejuvenation, 112–113
intense pulsed light (IPL), 4
    actinic keratoses PDT, 10, 48
    photorejuvenation, 10
    post-acne treatment, 19
    protoporphyrin IX activating dose, **5,** *5*
    skin rejuvenation, 102
intraepithelial neoplasia, 84
in vivo fluorescence monitoring, cutaneous T-cell lymphomas
    PDT, 92, *92, 93*
isotretinoin, sebaceous hyperplasia, 9

K

keratinocytic intraepidermal neoplasia (KIN), definition, 33

L

lactate dehydrogenase levels, ALA, *24*
lasers, 4
    acne PDT, 20–21
    skin cancer PDT, 71
Levulan
    actinic keratoses treatment, 8
        clinical trials, 38–39, **39,** 40, *41*
    costs, 43
    development, 1–2
    properties, **2**
    structure, *2*
lichen planus-like keratosis, 34
lichen planus PDT, 97
lichen sclerosis et atrophicus PDT, 96–97
lidocaine, actinic keratoses PDT, 60
light dose/intensity
    actinic keratoses PDT, 59
    cutaneous T-cell lymphomas PDT, 92
light-emitting diode devices
    acne PDT, 21, 23
    emission spectrum, *28*
    energy density, *28*
    skin cancer PDT, 71
light sources, 4–5
    acne PDT, 20–21
    actinic keratoses PDT, 59
    alternative light dosing, 4–5
    lasers, 4
    nonlaser, 4
    skin rejuvenation, 109
    warts PDT, 82–83
    see also specific types
long pulse dye laser/IPL, actinic keratoses PDT *see* actinic
    keratoses PDT

M

malignant melanoma metastases, PDT, 65
mechanism of action (PDT), 1, **1,** 89, *89*
melanocytes, photoaging, 102

metal halide lamps
    acne PDT, 21, *27*
    emission spectrum, *27*
    energy density, *28*
methotrexate, psoriasis therapy, 94
methylaminolevulinic acid (MALA)
    actinic keratoses PDT, 62
    BCC development in animal models, 55
    BCC PDT, 58
    clinical trials, 42
    development, 1–2
    properties, **2**
    skin penetration, 4
    skin rejuvenation, 109
    structure, *2*
Metvix, 10
    development, 1–2
    properties, **2**
    structure, *2*
microdermabrasion, pre-actinic keratoses PDT, 47, *47*
Mohs' surgery
    BCC, 8
    PDT adjuvant, 67

N

nausea, systemic ALA, 23
nevus sebaceous of Jadassohn, 9
nonporphyrins, as photosensitizers, 3
non-steroidal anti-inflammatory drugs (NSAIDs)
    actinic keratoses PDT, 49
    PDT contraindications, 70
    as photosensitizers, **108**

O

oral antioxidants, skin cancer prevention, 53
oral retinoids, skin cancer prevention, 53

P

p53 gene, BCC development, 56
pain
    psoriasis PDT, 96
    skin cancer PDT, 74
    warts PDT, **80,** 87–88
papulopustular lesions, acne PDT, 15–16, 19, *19, 21*
patient selection
    cutaneous T-cell lymphomas PDT, 90
    psoriasis PDT, 94
Pc 4, **2**
penetration enhancers, 67, 72
phenothiazines, as photosensitizers, **108**
photoaging, 101–102
    see also actinic keratoses; skin rejuvenation
Photochlor, **2**
Photocure lamp, warts PDT, 82–83
photodamage, ALA treatment, *6*
photofrin, 1
photorejuvenation *see* skin rejuvenation
photosensitizers, **2,** 2–3
    cytotoxicity mechanism, 2–3, **3**
    ideal properties, 2
    nonporphyrins, 3
    porphyrins, 3

photosensitizers (*cont'd*)
  skin rejuvenation, 107, 109
  systemic medications, **108**
  see also individual sensitizers
phototoxic reactions, skin rejuvenation, 111–112, *112*
phthalocyanine-4, **2**, 3
pigmentation, actinic keratoses, 34
porphobilinogen, formation, 3
porphyria, PDT contraindications, 70
porphyrins, as photosensitizers, 3
port wine stains, 99
pregnancy, PDT contraindications, 78
Propionibacterium acnes, 13–14
  see also acne
protoporphyrin IX (PpIX), 2
  absorption bands, 35–36, *36*
  actinic keratoses PDT, 35
  excitation spectrum, 20
  formation, 3
  light-activating dose, 4–5, **5,** *5*
psoralen in combination with ultraviolet radiation (PUVA), 61–62
  cutaneous T-cell lymphoma therapy, 90
  psoriasis therapy, 94
psoriasis
  alternative treatments, 94
  incidence, 94
psoriasis PDT, 94–96
  expected benefits, 94, *95*
  patient selection, 94
  side effects/complications, 96
  techniques, 94–96, **96**
    ALA concentrations, 94
    application times, 94
    multiple treatments, 95
    systemic *vs.* topical ALA, 95, 96
PTCH gene, BCC development, 55
pulsed-dye laser (PDL)
  port wine stain therapy, 97
  skin rejuvenation, 104–105
Purlytin, **2**
purpura, post-PDT, 44

R

race, ALA skin penetration, 3
radiotherapy
  BCC, 8, 66
  Bowen's disease, 8
  cutaneous T-cell lymphoma therapy, 90
red light sources
  actinic keratoses PDT, 37
  penetration, 66
retinoids, psoriasis therapy, 94

S

scarring, post-PDT, 44
scleroderma PDT, 97
sebaceous disorders, 9–10
  see also individual diseases/disorders
sebaceous glands
  ALA penetration, *14*
  PDT-ALA effects, 14–15, *17*
sebaceous hyperplasia, 9–10

seborrhea, 20
  treatment algorithm, *27*
'severe reactive acne,' acne PDT, *23*
singlet oxygen production, 1, **1**
skin cancer PDT, 65–76
  advantages, 74
  adverse effects, 74–75
  ALA, **75**
    MALA *vs.,* 72
  algorithm, *72, 72–74, 73, 74*
    tumor debulking, 71, 74
  alternative approaches, 74–75
  benefits, 67–68
    cosmesis, 75
  complications, 74–75
  light sources, 71
  MALA, **75**
    ALA *vs.,* 72
  Mohs' surgery adjuvant, 67
  pain management, 74
  patient interviews, 68
  patient selection, 67, **67**
  penetration enhancers, 67, 72
  photosensitizer application, 72
  surgery *vs.,* 74
  see also basal cell carcinoma (BCC) PDT; squamous cell
      carcinoma (SCC) PDT
skin cancer, prevention, 53–63
  see also actinic keratoses PDT
skin penetration
  ALA, 3, 4, *14, 15, 16*
    race/ethnicity, 3
  MALA, 4
skin preparation, actinic keratoses PDT, 47
skin rejuvenation, 10, 101–114, **102**
  algorithm, 109–110
  challenges, 102–103
  clinical trials, 103–105, **104**
  combination treatments, 103
  consent form, *107*
  cost analysis, 105
  expected benefits, 103–105, *106*
    actinic keratoses effects, 103
    Bowen's disease effects, 103
  incubation times, 109
  light sources, 109
    blue light PDT, 10
    coherent *vs.* noncoherent light sources, 105
    IPL, 10, *102*
  MALA, 109
  patient interviews, 105
  patient selection, 103, 105, 107
  photosensitizers, 107, 109
  post-treatment, 110–111
    active cooling, 110
    sunlight avoidance, 110–111, *112*
  pulsed-dye laser, 104–105
  side effects/complications, 111–112, *112–113*
    hyperpigmentation, 112
    hypopigmentation, 112
    infections, 112–113
    phototoxic reactions, 111–112, *112*

squamous cell carcinoma (SCC), 9, 53, 65
   actinic keratoses progression from, 7, 33, 34
      animal models, 54–55, *55, 56*
   conventional treatments, 9
   incidence, 53
squamous cell carcinoma (SCC) PDT, 9, 65, 72
   adverse effects, **7**
   treatment benefits, **7**
sulfonamides, as photosensitizers, **108**
sulfonylureas, as photosensitizers, **108**
sunlight avoidance, skin rejuvenation PDT, 110–111, 112
sunlight exposure, skin cancer, 53
sunscreens
   actinic keratoses PDT, 48–49
   skin cancer prevention, 53
surgery, skin cancer PDT *vs.*, 74
systemic 5-aminolevulinic acid (ALA), topical ALA *vs.*, 95, 96

T

tetracyclines, as photosensitizers, **108**
thiazide diuretics, as photosensitizers, **108**
tin etiopurpurin dichloride, **2,** 3
topical 5-FU, Bowen's disease, 8
topical 5-aminolevulinic acid (ALA), systemic ALA *vs.*, 95, 96
topical antioxidants, skin cancer prevention, 53
topical chemotherapy, actinic keratoses PDT, 49, **50**
topical retinoids, actinic keratoses PDT, **50**
topical vitamin D therapy, psoriasis therapy, 94
treatment tolerance, cutaneous T-cell lymphomas PDT, 92
tretinoin pretreatment, acne PDT, 20, 23
tricyclic antidepressants, as photosensitizers, **108**
tumor debulking, skin cancer PDT, 71, 74
tumor thickness, BCC PDT, 8

U

ultraviolet B radiation, psoriasis therapy, 94
ultraviolet examination, acne PDT, **14,** *18,* 18–19, *20*
uroporphyrinogen I, formation, 3

V

vascular lesions PDT, 97–98
Verteporfin, **2**
vitamin C iontophoresis, 19, 20, 29
   devices, *30*
   efficacy, *30*

W

warts, 77
   see also human papilloma virus (HPV)
warts, PDT
   active cooling, 87–88
   ALA *vs.* MALA, 81
   algorithm, 82, *82, 84*–86, 86–88
   alternative treatments, 87–88
   benefits, 78–79
      measurement, 78, **79**
   cost/benefit ratio, 79–81
   equipment, 82, *83*
   health insurance exclusion, 80–81
   light sources, 82–83
   patient selection, 78
   post-treatment care, 86–87
   recalcitrant, 80
   self-administration, 78, 83, 86
   side effects/complications, 87–88
      hyperpigmentation, 78–79
      pain, **80,** 87–88
wavelength (of light), tissue penetration, 2

X

xeroderma pigmentosum, 38